Communimetrics

John S. Lyons

Communimetrics

A Communication Theory of Measurement in Human Service Settings

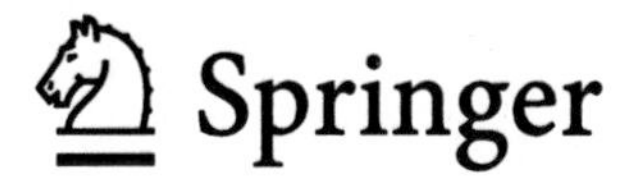

John S. Lyons
Endowed Chair of Child and Youth Mental Health Research
University of Ottawa and the Children's Hospital of Eastern Ontario
Canada

ISBN 978-0-387-92821-0 e-ISBN 978-0-387-92822-7
DOI 10.1007/978-0-387-92822-7
Springer Dordrecht Heidelberg London New York

Library of Congress Control Number: 2009926053

Printed on acid-free paper

Springer is part of Springer Science+Business Media (www.springer.com)

To Lise
The love of my life

Acknowledgments

The fact that I am the sole author of this book is exceptionally misleading. The experiences described herein involve a large number of individual, some of whose contributions simply cannot be underestimated.

My education started with Sally Bell Beck and Burton Woodruff at Butler University. Without their intervention I might have stayed in Chemistry. It continued at the graduate level with Nancy Hirschberg Wiggins and Alex Rosen as my primary mentors but a large number of other faculty at the University of Illinois at Chicago contributing to my intellectual development including Lee Wilkinson, Benjamin Kleinnuntz, Rowell Huessman, Leonard Eron, Chris Keys, Steven Reiss, Phil Friedman, and Harry Upshaw, in particular. Of course graduate school is also about peer support and I learned a great deal from my fellow students including Richard J. McNally, Howard Garb, Kim Mueser, Debra Brief, Wendy Epstein, Steve Sussman, Bruce McDonugh, Melissa Wattenberg, Robert Dolmetch, and Debbie Wintermuth. Postdoctoral studies were influenced by the privilege of studying at the University of Chicago with the scholarship of Donald W. Fiske, Benjamin Wright and Darrell Bach.

In my 24 years at Northwestern University I was influenced by a large number of colleagues, none more than Kenneth I. Howard who was my friend and mentor for nearly two decades. But, many others have had a significant impact on my professional and educational evolution including Richard Hughes, Sanford I. Finkel, Mark McGovern, Dana Weiner, Zoran Martinovich, Gene Griffin, Tracy Mallinson, Neil Jordan, Gary McClelland, among others.

I simply could not have completed this work without the tireless efforts of Laura Coats, Alison Schneider and Brandy Bedenfield. Ann LoPrieno has been a godsend in her contributions both to my work and Northwestern and the Praed Foundation.

One of the greatest blessings of working in a University setting is that you get the opportunity to teach but by teaching you learn more than you can imagine. Many of my graduate students have become my peers and I am grateful for what I have learned from them. I cherish my relationships with Dana Weiner, Purva Rawal, Cassandra Kisiel, Scott Leon, Dan Marston, Melissa Abraham, Matthew Shaw, Allison Ackerman, Dusty Humes. The same can be said for the postdoctoral fellows that I have had the privilege to mentor including Michael Jenuwine, Elizabeth Durkin, and Richard Epstein.

Scholars outside of Northwestern have always significantly contributed to the work inside this book. Frit Huyse has had a major impact on my professional development particularly in learning how to work collaboratively across multiple cultures. His Dutch colleagues Peter DeJonge, Brent Opmeer, Joris Slaets have also influenced the thinking behind this book. Ann Doucette whose knowledge and skills with regard to measurement are second to no one has helped me understand the relationship of communimetrics to other measurement theories. Rachel Anderson has been a tireless advocate and scholar in support of the approach. Robert Cohen has been a consistent voice of support and encouragement. Mike Cull, Kathy Gracey, and Richard Epstein have added to the work as have Gretchen Hall and Martha Henry.

And, all of the individuals working to help improve the lives of others who have embraced the use of measurement to achieve this goal are among the most important people to this story. I cannot name them all but they include Jess McDonald, Joseph Loftus, Patricia Chesler, Sue Ross, Brian Samuels, Tom Finnegan, Robert Wentworth, Randal Lea, Michael Leach, Betty Walton, Marcia Fazio, Allison Campbell, Erwin McEwen, Elyse Hart, Michael Rauso, Erika Tullberg, Susan Fry and many others. Betty Walton and Nathaniel Isread have made particularly important contributions.

At my new home at the University of Ottawa and the Children's Hospital of Eastern Ontario, I have already received support and encouragement to complete this work from Alex Mackenzie, Karen Tataryn, Simon Davidson, and Susan Richardson. My work with Stephanie Greenham, Janice Cohen, and Stephane Beaulne has informed this work.

Lise Bisnaire has been perhaps the most important personal and professional support that I have ever experienced in my life. Her consistent belief in the importance of my efforts and her ability to convert theory into practice in a fashion that directly helps children and families has been an inspiration. Words cannot fully describe my appreciation of her.

Contents

Chapter 1
Measurement in Human Service Enterprises: History and Challenges

After language our greatest invention is numbers.
—Benjamin Wright, 1997

Measurement is the foundation of the scientific enterprise. All major scientific breakthroughs were preceded by a revolution in measurement and instrumentation, the methods used to apply a measurement. However, measurement is not solely the purview of science. Measurement is also fundamental to commerce—you can't manage what you don't measure. Human service settings are often at the fulcrum between the scientific perspective, which informs practice, and the business perspective, which manages that practice. The emergence of the information age has ignited an enhanced interest in the use of measurement processes to inform the management of human services. However, the use of numbers in managing human affairs dates to antiquity. In the biblical story of Noah, God gave specific instructions on the dimensions of the arc that Noah was to build. Wright (1997) cites the Muslim rule of seven from Caliph 'Umar B. 'Abd al-'Aziz in Damacus in 723 AD. Taxes were not to exceed "seven weight." Similarly, the Magna Carta established uniform measurement of commodities and products such as wine, ale, and corn, throughout England (Runnymede, 1215 as cited in Wright, 1997). In large part, these measurement processes were intended to facilitate fairness and reduce conflict associated with disagreements in commerce. In fact, modern currency has its roots as a measurement strategy to equate the value of various goods and services. This measurement was not science, it was business. Now we are able to equate most currencies in the global marketplace, making trade easier even as these currencies fluctuate in relative value based on a host of complex factors. Consequently, although measurement is the foundation of science, to view measurement exclusively within the realm of normal science is limiting. Measurement also has a crucial role in commerce. Since human service enterprises are essentially a set of business models to apply scientifically acquired knowledge, it becomes necessary to simultaneously consider both the scientific and the commercial perspectives when applying measures.

Nunally (1976) describes measurement as consisting of "rules for assigning numbers to objects in such a way as to represent quantities of attributes" (p. 3). Numbers have the distinct advantage over words of being easily combined and manipulated. While Nunally's classic test was written for scientists, the goal of

J.S. Lyons, *Communimetrics: A Communication Theory of Measurement in Human Service Settings*,
DOI 10.1007/978-0-387-92822-7_1, © Springer Science+Business Media, LLC 2009

consistently assigning numbers to represent quantities of attributes is just as essential to all measurement, including business. Management based on objectives requires the ability to monitor the identified objectives, and subsequently measure those objectives (Drucker, 1954). At the simplest level, one cannot imagine a chief executive officer of a company remaining in that position for very long if the income from product sales consistently did not exceed the costs of producing the product and taking it to market. To compete effectively in a competitive marketplace, businesses have grown more quality conscious. One could not imagine an automobile factory that kept building cars that won't start and don't move. All automobile producers test drive their cars. Nor could one imagine a winery not keeping count of the number of bottle, cases, and casks produced and sold. And, of course, wineries routinely taste test their products before sale.

Instrumentation facilitates the effective use of measurement in both science and commerce. Advancing in instrumentation to measure brain activity, such as positron emission tomography (PET) and functional magnetic resonance imaging (fMRI) has revolutionized this area of research and improved medical practice. Improved inventory control methods allow just-in-time management in grocery stores and other retail businesses to improve efficiency, reduce waste, and improve profitability.

Sometimes, however, we wish to measure things that are not readily accessible to instrumentation. Particularly in human service enterprises, the objectives of service delivery are often more difficult to describe and measure. For example, a program for homeless individuals that attempts to find housing can readily measure whether the individual has a place to live. Whether that place feels safe and comfortable to the individual is not as easy to assess. Often the objective of a service system involves characteristics of people that are not easily accessible to instrumentation, and are, therefore, more difficult to measure. Due, in part, to this limitation, human services are one of the last sectors of our economy to fully embrace the application of measurement processes to its work. Most industries routinely apply measurement processes to ensure quality and inform management decisions. While attention to quality in human services has a history over the past four decades, it is not the case that the actual goals and objectives of most human services are routinely measured and managed. A program may measure the number of people served or the units of service provided, but they do not routinely measure the impact of those services on the lives of those served. This historical reality, however, is beginning to change.

Most measurement in the human service settings has been done on an atheoretical, ad hoc basis. The measurement of age or gender does not require a theory or a complicated measurement operation. Many pieces of information—admission/enrollment date, time of service, disposition—do not require formal theories of measurement. This convenience of measurement has had two unintended consequences. First, if this is the only information available to managers, they will manage these numbers only. Second, the science of studying human service enterprises frequently relies on convenience databases, so most services research has focused on these easy-to-measure constructs, as they are readily available and trustworthy in large service databases.

However, there are many things that influence the human service delivery processes that are more complicated. In medicine and behavioral health, there is the clinical presentation, i.e., symptoms and signs of illness. In vocational rehabilitation, there are issues of job skills and capacities. In services for individuals with developmental disability, there are the constructs of adaptive functioning. For business incubation, there are characteristics of the business plan and capacity of the entrepreneur. All of these constructs require some forethought to create formal operations that result in their reliable and valid measurement.

Over the past several decades in the human service setting, measurement is beginning to transcend its traditional role as a component of the scientific enterprise to assume a role in the management of programs and systems. Management strategies focused on monitoring the success of achieving specific objectives (e.g., Behn, 2003) have grown in popularity in all business sectors, human services included. In order to better understand the evolving role of measurement in human services settings, it is useful to first consider the business environment of these settings.

Differences Between Measurement in Science and Commerce

In the physical sciences there is a remarkable consistency with which core constructs are measured. Factors such as weight, specific mass, speed, and temperature have all remained fairly constant, albeit with some significant advances in instrumentation and occasional retooling of the metrics used to express values. However, even when changed these metrics have direct translations from one to the other. That is, 32°F is exactly 0°C. Similarly, miles per hour can be consistently translated into meters per second without forcing a reconsideration of either measurement.

While commerce shares many common precepts for measurement with science, it is also true that measurement in commerce is very much bound by the nature of the marketplace. For example, album sales used to be the universal metric for the success of an artist's popular appeal in the music industry. This metric worked well when vinyl records were the unit sold. The metric continued its utility when the industry standard shifted from vinyl to compact discs. But, in the past few years, the music industry has changed again, this time to digitalized music, which can be sent across the Internet in any variety of packages. Now industry leaders talk in terms of the number of "downloads" to capture the same construct of which artist has the most popular music. Downloads cannot be readily translated back into album sales.

Measurement is further complicated by cultural factors. Good measurement in science is intended to be free of cultural influences. These factors are thought of within the framework of measurement error—things that make the measurement less likely to be accurate. In counterpoint, good measurement in commerce is much more likely to be dependent on cultural factors. Like record sales, abandoned measurement frameworks litter the history of business.

A second way in which measurement is different in commerce is that it must be far more accessible. The number of individuals who need to be able to understand a measure in commerce is a far larger population than that for most scientific measurements. The results of the measurement process are widely communicated in commerce. In fact, one could argue that the results of measurement become the language of the marketplace (e.g., number of threads in a sheet, carats in a diamond). For this reason, a good measure must be simpler to express and easier to understand by a wide range of participants in the marketplace. In science, measurement needs only be understood by fellow scientists to allow replication.

To better appreciate the role of measurement in commerce it is useful to understand the variability in types of markets. Gilmore and Pine (1997) described what they called the hierarchy of offerings to inventory, in order of complexity, different things that could be sold in a marketplace. The five types of offering, starting with the least complicated:

1. *Commodities*. Raw materials such as oil and grain
2. *Products*. Offerings produced from commodities. Gasoline is made from oil. Cereal is made from grain
3. *Services*. Hiring someone to apply a product for you; activities with defined outcomes performed for others, i.e., getting your clothes dry cleaned, your car washed, getting a passport
4. *Experiences*. Memories; activities in which part of the outcome is the process by which the activity is provided, i.e., going to the theater or an amusement park
5. *Transformation*. Notable personal change resulting from the activity or intervention, i.e., health/fitness program, behavioral health services

As you go higher on the hierarchy of offerings, the measurements and measurement processes necessary to support management become more complex. Commodities are measured in quantities such as weight and volume, and higher-order qualities such as purity. This is the lowest level offering and the simplest to measure.

Products are measured in quantities such as units, and qualities such as durability and attractiveness. Products are intended to be available to everyone. How many were sold? How quickly were they delivered? Did they work? Did they last long enough for the consumer to be satisfied? Of course, there is also measurement on the production side. How many units were produced? At what cost? How quickly could they be shipped and distributed? To where are they distributed?

Services are measured in quantities often in units of time and qualities such as timeliness and consumer satisfaction. Drying cleaning, construction, and painting all are services. You hire somebody to apply a product for you because either you don't have the time or the expertise to do it yourself. How many people were served? Did they come back? Would they recommend this service to a friend? Were they happy with the result? On the production side, the focus of measurement of services is often on the productivity of service staff, the cost per unit service, and the availability to service capacity to meet demand.

Experiences begin to become a bit more complicated from a measurement perspective. Here the primary offering is the creation of a meaningful memory. High-quality funeral homes offer a range of services (e.g., the preparation of the deceased for burial or cremation), but they also offer an experience (e.g., the opportunity for the bereaved friends and families to mourn their lost loved one in a warm, caring, and dignified way). Amusement parks offer a mix of services (e.g., food, drink) and experiences (e.g., thrill rides). Experiences are almost exclusively measured in terms of consumer satisfaction. Did you like it? Do you think you will come back? Did you come back? Would you send a friend? Of course, on the production side, issues such as safety and costs are important considerations for measurement.

Transformations require the most complex measurement of any market. A transformational offering is one designed to provide the opportunity for an individual to change personally in some important way. Education is the most widespread transformational offering. The purpose of most educational offerings is to change the student or participant's knowledge or even perspective on particular content areas (e.g., math, language, leadership). In order to assess the impact of education, it is generally necessary to determine what a person knew prior to the educational offering. Thus, in order to measure transformations, you are required to measure a change in status that occurs over time. The measurement of change within an individual is enormously more complicated from both a measurement perspective and the process of collecting, analyzing, and interpreting the measurement process than that required for the first four offerings.

While many human service enterprises are interested in the customer's experience, the experience per se is seldom the actual offering. More likely, these enterprises are offering either services (e.g., driver's licenses) or transformations (e.g., recovery from addiction, housing stabilization, improvement in functioning). It is the last offering that necessitates a new way of thinking about the management of these enterprises. If the goal of the enterprise is merely to assist others in the application of a product, i.e., provide a service, management need only focus on whether that goal was accomplished satisfactorily. However, if the goal of the enterprise is to actually facilitate a change process, it is necessary to measure that which may or may not change if one is to manage offerings in a transformational marketplace. Many, but not all, human service enterprises are transformational offerings. They exist to promote change in those served.

If most human service enterprises are transformational offerings and you cannot manage what you do not measure, then it becomes incumbent upon human services administrations to develop the capacity to monitor the potential transformational effects of their enterprise. It is this realization that naturally leads to an increase in efforts to assess and manage outcomes within this business sector. Thus, the business of helping people requires the measurement of how people change. Measurement of change in humans becomes a central component of managing systems designed to help them. This book uses the general term *human service enterprises* rather than *human services*, to remind the reader that we are often not measuring services; rather, we are measuring enterprises intended to serve humans. With an understanding that human service enterprises are often transformational offerings, it is useful to explore a brief history of measurement as it informs our work in this field.

The History and Definition of Measurement

Much of what we know about the theory of measurement comes from the scientific tradition. Sir Francis Galton (1822–1911) is generally credited with the first measurement of a psychological construct. He coined the term *biometry* to describe his efforts to measure such things as intelligence. He believed that intelligence was related to the keenness of one's sense; therefore, he developed tests of sensory acuity using reaction time and other procedures. He also pioneered the concepts of correlation and regression to study the relationship between measures. His basic measurement approach was to apply instrumentation to processes that he posited to be related to psychological constructs. Current intelligence testing continues to adhere to this basic measurement approach. Similarly, Galton pioneered fingerprint matching by establishing a set of measurement procedures to be applied to a fingerprint. Matching is done on the profile of these measures, not the fingerprint itself. This method is still in use today.

As mentioned, Nunally (1976), in his classic book on psychometrics, defines measurement as consisting of "rules for assigning numbers to objects in such as way as to represent quantities of attributes" (p. 3). The rules by which numbers are assigned are the foundation of measurement. Those rules are generally established based on the objectives of the measurement process and guided by a theory of measurement. He further specifies the following advantages of standardized measurement:

- *Objectivity*. Through objectivity a statement of fact made by one person can be verified by another.
- *Quantification*. Assigning numbers to observations has two advantages. First, it allows a finer detailed description than would be possible otherwise. Second, it allows different observations to be combined thus creating an ability to aggregate experiences.
- *Communication*. "Science is a highly public enterprise in which efficient communication among scientists is essential" (p. 7).
- *Economy*. Standardized measurement is generally less expensive than individualized assessments that often take longer and are less consistent.
- *Scientific Generalization*. Measurement allows us to move beyond a single set of observations to create an understanding of a broader range of experiences.

All five of these characteristics of measurement are directly relevant to human service systems. However, two of these have far greater implications than imagined when measurement is the sole province of scientists. First, economy is critical in that the measurement itself becomes part of the business enterprise, and any expense involved in the measurement becomes a part of the cost of supplying the intervention. Second, while Nunally is absolutely correct about the importance of communication in science, in human service applications, the nature of communication expands geometrically. Communication no longer occurs just among scientists. The need for communication also applies once you enter the marketplace.

You cannot have a scientist come in and perform and interpret all measurement operations. That would be absurd. Everyone in the human service delivery enterprise must be engaged in the measurement process. And everyone in that process has the inherent right to understand that measurement process and any implications of a specific measurement result. In human services enterprises, the use of measurement is similar to the use of money. Everyone in the market needs to understand the relative value of the currency. Markets do not work effectively if one person does not understand the currency. In transformational offerings, all parties have to understand the transformation in order for the market to work effectively.

The next major innovation in measurement was Feinstein's (1987) contribution, *clinimetrics*, which recognizes the increasingly important role of the communication aspects of measurement in medical settings. His book begins with "Like Moliere's bourgeois gentleman who was astonished to discover that he spoke in prose, patients and clinicians may not realize that they constantly communicate with clinimetric indexes" (p. 1). Clinimetrics remains predominantly a scientific enterprise as a method for describing the clinical status of human factors not readily measurable with instrumentation. A major shift in clinimetrics was that the measurement approach was designed to support the clinical judgment aspects of combining inputs from multiple inputs to generate the measurement of a construct (Feinstein).

Over the past century, psychometric theory and clinimetrics have resulted in an explosion in the number of measures that have been developed and used in various human service settings. In behavioral health alone, Lambert, Ogles, and Masters (2000) identified more than 1,400 different published measures. If you were to combine across all human service settings, the number of different measures is enormous.

Problems that Result from the Development of Measures by Normal Science

Given the staggering number of measures already in existence and the large body of research and debate about measurement theories, including psychometrics and clinimetrics, what is the justification for a new theory of measurement for the human services setting? With all of these approaches there remain fundamental problems that limit their utility. The first problem arises from the context of science. The ethics of the scientific enterprise require informed consent and confidentiality of responses. Thus, respondents in survey type measurement process are told that the results will have no implications for their lives and will be held in strict confidence. This procedure is both thought to protect the rights of the subjects or scientific experiments and also to remove any motivation for providing misleading information. In other words, confidentiality and irrelevance to action are thought to increase respondents' likelihood of telling the truth. That philosophy represents a completely different context compared with respondents' experience in human service settings.

With the exception of anonymous consumer satisfaction surveys completed after all services and interventions are complete, most measurement in these contexts is done for the express purpose of assisting decision making relevant to the people in the service transaction. In fact, the measurement process is a form of communication among parties in the transaction. It is inherently influenced by all of the contingencies that might affect that transaction.

Second, while clinimetric measurement often focuses on the measure of a single construct, most measurement processes involve the use multiple inputs (e.g., questions) to create scale scores by summing or average over a set of items. The major challenge with this strategy is that the resultant value (e.g., scale score) is at least one step removed from the responses, and scale scores can be hard to interpret. What does a score of 30 mean? How does it compare with a 17? There has been significant effort to increase the interpretability of scale scores by converting them into common metrics. This goal is generally accomplished through a technique called *norming* the data. The most common example are T scores, in which the mean is 50 and standard deviation is 10. However, interpreting a T score still requires some understanding of the mean and standard deviation. And, of course, generating normative data actually requires that we have the population mean and standard deviation.

It is certainly possible to educate large populations to be able to apply measurement scales. Most people in the United States are able to understand the meaning of 60°F and its difference from 30°F. Most other countries use the Centigrade scale, with similar success of the population understanding the temperatures. Of course, Americans traveling in Canada or Europe may take some time before they are able to convert temperatures that they hear in Centigrade into something they understand. Similarly, the use of IQ as a common metric of intelligence is a relatively successful cross-cultural communication, although with nowhere near the widespread use of temperature. Regardless, the overall number of common metrics we can anticipate the population to be able to fully understand is probably relatively small. Thus, easy interpretation is an unmet need in most measurement processes, particularly when measurement ventures outside of the scientific community. In fact, depending on how one is managing the enterprise, it may be desirable to have everyone in the market system be familiar with a given measure.

Measurement as Communication

If one accepts the assertion that in human service enterprises the relative value of communication exceeds the relative value of other principles of measurement and that the nature of communication in these settings is substantially broader than communication in science, what implications does that have for a theory of measurement? It is the premise of this book that reconsidering measurement from a communication perspective results in a rethinking of many of the underlying premises upon which traditional measurement approaches have been constructed.

In understanding this reformulation of measurement, perhaps it is best to begin with a brief overview of the field of communication.

Communication Theory and Measurement

The field of communication is broad and diverse, and is often organized along disciplinary lines and struggles to share common theories and approaches (Anderson, 1996). Donsbach (2006), in his presidential address to the Annual Conference of the International Communication Association, argues that communications lacks an identified "object" that even allows it to be considered a field. Although most universities have programs that focus on aspects of communications, these programs' foci vary dramatically from one place to the next. While the nature of the field is overwhelmingly pluralistic, it is also the case that a substantial body of knowledge exists—often strictly within disciplines (e.g., psychology, sociology). While I will not attempt to exhaustively review the field as it applies to human services enterprises, there is a body of literature that is particularly relevant to our discussion.

One of the early models of communication that is most relevant to measurement in service delivery settings may be the transmission concept. This model has been dated back to the eighteenth-century British Empiricists (Peters, 1989). In this way of thinking, communication is the process by which information is transferred from one person's mind to that of another (e.g., Rothenbuhler, 1998). It is the process by which a message is sent and received. Thus, the study of communication focuses on how information is created and packaged and sent and then received and processed—much like understanding the postal service. Letters are considered, written, addressed, mailed, delivered, received, opened, read, and understood by a second party.

This example of a linear process of information transfer is becoming increasingly quaint. While the example of a letter was a common experience congruent with the communication theories of the time, today most 18 year olds may not have even written, let alone mailed, a letter. New forms of communication such as e-mail, texting, and instant messaging have reduced our reliance on letters as a form of communication. These new communication options also reveal the limits of transmission theories of communication.

It is worth noting that the transmission model of communication is congruent with the generic model of psychotherapy outcomes proposed by Howard, Kipta, Krause, and Orlinsky (1986). As shown in Figure 1.1, in this general model of understanding mental health services, three components of the process are considered—input, throughout, and output.

Using this general concept, the authors' then discuss how to study components at each of the three stages of the process. Input characteristics include client and

INPUT → THRUPUT → OUTPUT

Fig. 1.1 A general model of understanding mental health services

provider characteristics and geographic considerations. Throughput characteristics include the nature of the treatment approach, the development of a therapeutic bond (i.e., the quality and strength of the relationship between the therapist and client), and dose (i.e., the number of sessions of therapy received). And output characteristics refer to outcomes from the therapeutic process that include such things as remoralization, symptom relief, and functional improvement, and also therapist reimbursement, consumer satisfaction, and future referrals of friends and acquaintances to the therapist. The linear process described in the generic model is consistent with the linear construction of the transmission models of communication. The limitations are the same. The model does not have a mechanism to describe any impact that throughput or output processes might have on input characteristics. For example, referrals to a particular therapist often come from satisfied clients of that therapist who have friends or acquaintances seeking help.

Although still a popular theoretical approach, recently transmission models have come to be viewed as conceptually flawed by some theorists. Transmission models tend to be simplistically linear in that they view information as only moving from point A to point B and struggle to include inputs from point B that might actually change the nature of information coming from point A (Carey, 1989). Several theorists (e.g., Deetz, 1994; Pearce, 1989; Shepherd, 1993) have proposed a constitutive model that conceptualizes communication as a meaning making activity. In this view communication is a process that produces and reproduces shared meaning. This conceptual model of communication has a great deal of utility for measurement in human service enterprises as the goal of assessment (read measurement) processes can be thought to be the development of a shared meaning between the recipient and the provider with regard to actual service needs.

The shift in priority of the measurement process toward the meaning-making value of the measurement changes the focus of the measurement process away from a focus on the application of a specific measurement procedure to the observation of an individual. The construction of the measure is all about ensuring that the observation is replicable (i.e., high reliability) and accurate (i.e., high validity). When you consider a constitutive perspective, the focus shifts away from the procedure used to observe, or the inputs of the process, to the procedures use to share the results of the measurement process—to communicate—the output of the measurement process. Figure 1.2 provides a graphic illustration of the basic focal difference between traditional measurement approaches and the use of measurement to communicate; that is, communimetrics.

This figure graphically suggests that the priorities of measurement under communimetrics are different than under traditional approaches to measurement. The emphasis of measurement is on its value for communicating thoughts and observations within an enterprise. The primary reason to measure within the enterprise is to communicate to someone else either on behalf of an individual served or for program or system aggregates (i.e., summaries of individuals served). Therefore, why not create the measurement process to optimize the communication utility of the measure? In fact, why not reconceptualize measurement in these settings entirely? Ben Wright said that after language, numbers are our greatest invention.

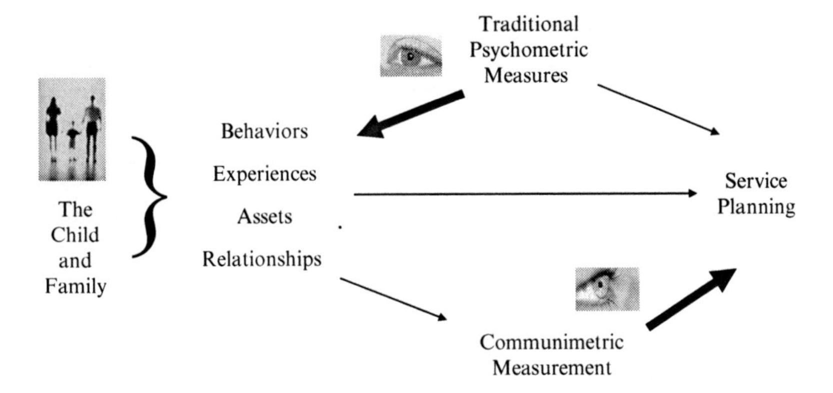

Fig. 1.2 A graphic illustration of the basic focal difference between traditional measurement approaches and the use of measurement to communicate

I would argue that numbers are actually a unique form of language that allows its aggregation. In this way of thinking, numbers are the first common language.

Communimetrics and the Philosophy of Science

Most traditional measurement approaches have their philosophy of science embedded in empiricist traditions of logical positivism and related philosophies dating back to the eighteenth century. Logical empiricism (positivism) has been described as the received epistemology of psychology from its origins to the 1960s (Capaldi & Proctor, 2000). The major tenet of logical empiricism is that all knowledge is based on logical inferences from observable facts. The historical context of the rise of logical empiricism was post-World War I Europe and a struggle for science to transcend theology and metaphysics. While there are many variations within logical empiricisms, one of its strongest tenets is that a proposition is only meaningful if there exists a finite procedure for verifying whether it is true or false (Hempel, 1950). Popper (1959) famously criticized the logical empiricists focus on verifiability, stating that such a goal was impossible and shifted it to falsifiability. In other words, conceptually, it had to be possible to prove if it could ever be consider it to be true.

Both major psychometric theories, classical test theory and item response theory, have their philosophical basis in logical empiricism. The principle is that measurement is the application of a "finite procedure" to exact a verifiable (or falsifiable) truth from an observation. Implicit in measurement theory is the concept that some real phenomenon exists that science is attempting to measure—a truth revealed by the measurement process. A fundamental difference between measurement under the theory of communimetrics and traditional measurement theory is that communimetrics makes no assumption that one is divining the "truth" about what is being observed through the measurement process. One is only attempting to communicate what he or she thinks is true at any given time.

This absence of a requirement of an underlying "truth" separate from the observation is a fundamental difference with traditional measurement. The task of measurement in communimetrics is to describe what one believes to be true. Whether or not the result of a measurement operation, in fact, is representing some independently verifiable (or falsifiable) objective reality is not the primary goal of this measurement process. That is not to stay that some absolute truth does not exist; nor that in an ideal application that a communimetric measure would not capture such realities. Communimetrics simply takes no opinion on this important issue in the philosophy of science. In other words, it does not take an ontological perspective. Regardless of whether and what truth exists, we continue to need to communicate about what we see, believe, think, and desire in order to survive in a social world. In communimetrics, measurement is describing what one believes that one knows, or perhaps more accurately, what one knows that one believes. Whether one, in fact, does know it or not, or even whether it is something that is knowable, is immaterial to the process of communimetric measurement itself.

One could make the argument that communimetrics attempts to measure the construct of the common (or shared) truth. That is, a logical empiricist philosophy could still be applied, but the phenomenon is not the construct named in the item but rather the shared belief about the level of the item among participants in the measurement process. For example, a communimetric tool for children's behavioral health does not measure oppositional behavior per se. Instead, it measures the common understanding of a specific child's behavior toward authority relative to the beliefs of the parties involved in completing the assessment tool. In this way, communimetrics is not necessarily incongruent with logical positivist tenets and traditions, but neither does it rest upon them.

It is also possible that communimetrics can be seen as consistent with a relativist perspective (e.g., Kuhn, 1962). In his classic, *The Structure of Scientific Revolutions*, Kuhn posited that science was predominantly a social enterprise and that scientists would agree on a shared understanding that would define normal science for a period. New scientists would present information that would change this "social construction" of normal science periodically in what Kuhn would call a paradigm shift. In this model, there is no real progress, only periodic "palace coups" replacing old science with new. Perhaps even more to the point, instrumentalists such as Toulmin (1970) might argue that language is a game in which notions of truth and falsehood are irrelevant. In this framework, all meaning depends on the perspective from which the instrumentation is applied. The creation of a shared meaning through a measurement process is certainly consistent with aspects of the relativist perspective. It is, in fact, a social construction. Of course in the absence of *any* notion of truth or falsehood of meaning, concepts such as reliability and validity of measures are at least overwhelmingly complex and, at worse, moot. In a completely relativistic word even the concept of a common language is meaningless.

More recently, philosophers have attempted to bridge the enormous gap between logical positivist and social constructionists by attempting to blend useful aspects from both philosophies into an integrated approach that recognizes both the opportunity to seek truth and real progress through science and that the process of science is an inherently social and political activity (e.g., Manicas, 2006).

Manicas (2006) states that the goal of science is both explanation and understanding, not necessarily prediction. He further clarifies that the difference between natural and social sciences involve consciousness and that the social scientist is a part of the reality that he or she investigates. According to this theory, the primary goal of the social scientist is to clarify the social mechanisms that allow people to structure, but not determine outcomes. This approach allows for the distortions that arise from the social and political influences in social sciences without fully giving in to them as the essence of science. This theoretical stance is referred to as reality theory, suggesting its realistic approach to the limitation of science place on it being a human enterprise.

At the conceptual edge of the reality theory school of thought, Laudan's (1990) concept of normative naturalism provides an integrative alternative to the extremes of positivism and relativism. In fact, Laudan would not even view empiricism and relativism as always on the opposite ends of the same continuum. In his view, they share a number of common assumptions. His application of pragmatic arguments leads to a more realistic evaluation of theory and measurement.

Pavin (1999) has attempted to integrate the scientific realism philosophy of science into communication theory in what he calls *the third way* (neither empiricism nor relativism). According to this author, acceptance of a realist philosophy into communications requires three different commitments:

- To the reality of one's theoretical concepts
- To scientific explanation as a causal process
- To the reliability of meaning

The first commitment to the reality of one's theoretical concepts implies that theories are not component parts that can be constructed and deconstructed based on new findings. The proliferation of different words to describe the same phenomenon has been a source of confusion in the social sciences. From a realist perspective, if all relevant causal processes do not vary across different terms, then these terms are exactly the same thing. If many of the causal processes are invariant, then differently named constructs may represent overlapping phenomenon.

The case of post-traumatic stress disorder (PTSD) is an interesting and potentially controversial case in point (APA, 2004). Table 1.1 presents the current diagnostic criteria used in DSM-IVTR to define this diagnosis. First, included in the formal nosology of psychiatric disorders in the third version of DSM (APA, 1980), Trimble (1985) traces the history of the phenomenon covered in this diagnosis back hundreds of years. One of the historical examples Trimble uses includes a description of Samuel Pepys' diary regarding his nightmares following the great fire of London. Some of the experience Pepys records can be found listed in Table 1.1. Of course in Pepys' time, there was no name for his experience.

Table 1.1 Diagnostic criteria for Post-Traumatic Stress Disorder (PTSD)

A. "The person has been exposed to a traumatic event in which both of the following were present:
   (1) the person experienced, witnessed, or was confronted with an event or events that involved actual or threatened death or serious injury, or a threat to the physical integrity of self or others
   (2) the person's response involved intense fear, helplessness, or horror. Note: In children, this may be expressed instead by disorganized or agitated behavior

B. The traumatic event is persistently re-experienced in one (or more) of the following ways:
   (1) recurrent and intrusive distressing recollections of the event, including images, thoughts, or perceptions. Note: In young children, repetitive play may occur in which themes or aspects of the trauma are expressed.
   (2) recurrent distressing dreams of the event. Note: In children, there may be frightening dreams without recognizable content.
   (3) acting or feeling as if the traumatic event were recurring (includes a sense of reliving the experience, illusions, hallucinations, and dissociative flashback episodes, including those that occur on awakening or when intoxicated). Note: In young children, trauma-specific reenactment may occur.
   (4) intense psychological distress at exposure to internal or external cues that symbolize or resemble an aspect of the traumatic event
   (5) physiological reactivity on exposure to internal or external cues that symbolize or resemble an aspect of the traumatic event

C. Persistent avoidance of stimuli associated with the trauma and numbing of general responsiveness (not present before the trauma), as indicated by three (or more) of the following:
   (1) efforts to avoid thoughts, feelings, or conversations associated with the trauma
   (2) efforts to avoid activities, places, or people that arouse recollections of the trauma
   (3) inability to recall an important aspect of the trauma
   (4) markedly diminished interest or participation in significant activities
   (5) feeling of detachment or estrangement from others
   (6) restricted range of affect (e.g., unable to have loving feelings)
   (7) sense of a foreshortened future (e.g., does not expect to have a career, marriage, children, or a normal life span)

D. Persistent symptoms of increased arousal (not present before the trauma), as indicated by two (or more) of the following:
   (1) difficulty falling or staying asleep
   (2) irritability or outbursts of anger
   (3) difficulty concentrating
   (4) hypervigilance
   (5) exaggerated startle response

E. Duration of the disturbance (symptoms in Criteria B, C, and D) is more than 1 month.

F. The disturbance causes clinically significant distress or impairment in social, occupational, or other important areas of functioning.

   Specify if:
   Acute: if duration of symptoms is less than 3 months
   Chronic: if duration of symptoms is 3 months or more

   Specify if:
   With Delayed Onset: if onset of symptoms is at least 6 months after the stressor" pp 467-468

From American Psychiatric Association (2004). Diagnostic and Statistical Manual of Mental Disorder 4th Edition Text Revision (DSM-IV TR). Washington, DC: American Psychiatric Association Press.

Among the names used to describe individuals' intense reactions to extremely adverse life events include symptoms proposed to be caused by experiences in warfare, including shell shock, battle fatigue, battle neurosis, combat exhaustion, and post-traumatic neurosis (Trimble, 1985). Myers (1940) famously analyzed the experiences of 2,000 war veterans and attempted to distinguish what he referred to as *shell shock* and *shell concussion*. The latter was caused by exploding missiles. The former was proposed to be caused by horror and terror. Similar phenomena were described for adverse events that did not involve warfare. Rigler (1879 as cited in Trimble, 1985) proposed the concept of compensation neurosis to describe the impact on disability reports following railway accidents once compensation laws were passed. Nervous shock was proposed to describe some of the psychological sequelae following accidents (Page, 1885). Miller (1961 as cited in Trimble, 1987) used the term accident neurosis. More recently Kijak and Funtowicz (1982) proposed the survivor syndrome to capture psychological reactions to disaster experiences.

As McNally (2004) discusses, PTSD as a formal diagnostic category was included in DSM-III, in part due to sociopolitical considerations to find a psychiatric disorder that covered the symptoms experienced by returning veterans of the Vietnam War. There is substantial debate within and without the mental health field about the syndromic validity of the diagnostic category PTSD. When it was first proposed many psychiatrists felt the symptoms were already covered by existing psychiatric disorders (e.g., phobias and other anxiety disorders). Currently, many traumatologists see any questioning of the syndrome as politically motivated. Currently, there is a movement among child psychiatrists to push for a shift in the syndrome to allow for a better description of children who have symptoms resulting from adverse experiences (Developmental Trauma; Cook et al., 2005; van der Kolk, 2005). Even what constitutes a traumatic experience became subject to debate as the other advocates attempted to utilize the success of the PTSD label for creating help for Vietnam veterans to serve their own causes. The one sure result we can take from the ongoing debates about trauma and its impact is that we will be calling the phenomenon something different in the not-too-distant future. Regardless, there is something real there. There is no doubt that when people experience extreme and life-threatening life events, it has psychological ramifications.

Despite the variety of names to label the phenomena and efforts to differentiate components, there is an underlying reality that nearly everyone agrees exists—when humans experience extreme events the psychological consequences frequently include anxiety, avoidance, uncontrolled remembering, and sleep-related problems. The job of science is to resolve the controversies about cause and effect in a fashion that clarifies etiology and treatment. However, in the meantime, people who work in the mental health service delivery system need to use what we think we know now to attempt to do the best we can to help. We can't wait for science to resolve all debates before we try to help people today. Thus, using consensus-developed communication strategies based on ideas and theoretical constructs that are believed to be real at the present time is a relevant requirement of a communication-based theory of measurement. We do not need to assume an underlying truth to have a useful and meaningful consensus communication, but that does not mean that an underlying truth is not actually there. We leave that for the march of science to resolve.

The second commitment is to the goal of science as determining causal processes rather than predicting observed events. According to realist philosophy of science, the very nature of the scientific endeavor is to build an understanding of the structures and processes underlying events that determine the natural relationships among these events. This commitment means that measures that build in cause-and-effect models might be less stable than those that allow science to continue to clarify cause-and-effect relationships. Measurement might best focus on the components in this model rather than assuming causal relationships among components.

The final commitment is the one most directly relevant to measurement as communication, and that is the commitment to the reality of meaning. Pavin (1999) distinguishes between meaning and significance. "Meaning is a socially shared characteristic of language; significance is an individually unique response to language" (p. 183). A major implication of this perspective is that meaning is reliable. Multiple observers take the same meaning from a communication.

A desire exists to get at the truth. Most physicians, psychologists, social workers, child welfare workers, or business executives believe that there are basic realities to their situations as they apply to the nature of their enterprises. However, the assessment of these basic realities among the people served by these enterprises is accomplished in an open system that is invariably fraught with complexities from the relative value of competing and contradictory information from different sources to the financial incentives for different measurement results. As such, the conceptualization of measurement must consider these complicating factors in order to achieve what everyone agrees upon as the goal—accurate and meaningful information about the people served. The realist notion of referential realism is a key to the success of measurement as communication (e.g., Schwartz, 1977). We may not fully understand the "true meaning" to which an item refers but we can still fully understand what that item is intended to mean.

Science sometimes can catch up to communication. Pavin (1999) uses the history of water to illustrate this point. English speakers talked about *water* and constructively used the term, while Spanish speakers used the term *aqua* and French speakers spoke of *eau*. These words were widely used to successfully communicate for centuries before scientists learned that the best was to actually characterize water was as a chemical compound with two parts hydrogen and one part oxygen, H_2O. This discovery did not render irrelevant the communications about water/aqua/eau that occurred before the scientific consensus regarding H_2O. These terms had referential realism that was then confirmed by scientific investigation. It would seem silly to me to propose, consistent with relativist theories, that the word water/aqua/eau was simply a set of convenient fictions.

Numbers were created, in part, as a means to identify and communicate a common standard. Measurement was created to establish and communicate rules for assigning numbers to accomplish the goal of a common standard. But one also can reverse this process. The process of defining numbers through measurement can be used to build a consensus around how to describe things. Once a measurement process is in place it can help further communications about the phenomenon measured. Further, organizing existing communications through the assignment of numbers can facilitate our communication by allowing the aggregation process available to numbers that simply do not exist for other forms of language. The very process of establishing procedures for measurement of a common standard can then be used to establish and apply that common standard. In human service enterprises, measurement as communication is not a linear process. It is more of a conceptual dialog between that which is to be measured and those who seek to measure. The recognition of the nonlinearity of the measurement process in no way forces us to deny the reality of the construct sought to measure. Rather, it accepts that as humans our ability to understand complex phenomena is a fluid process facilitated by experience and feedback. It simply recognizes and integrates the interactive and iterative aspects of human learning into the measurement process.

Communimetric measurement is by definition subjective. Merriam-Webster's third definition of subjective is: "a: characteristic of or belonging to reality as perceived rather than as independent of mind." These measures are designed to reflect the output of a thinking process. They can never be fully independent of the mind that was used to create them. Measurement from this perspective is a judgment. Communimetrics is designed to make thinking processes transparent and provide a conceptual organization or framework for the thinkers to be attuned to the relevant factors that must be thought through in any particular circumstance. Despite the fact communimetric measures reflect judgments, they still can be reliable. There are common practices, understandings, and realities in human service enterprises that everyone can learn to identify and describe.

My personal experiences in measurement have influenced my perception of the value of global ratings informed by those who are working directly with people. Like everyone else with a Ph.D., I received my doctorate, in part, based on the completion of a dissertation. I was trained in the late 1970s and early 1980s, which were halcyon days for behavioral assessment strategies. Although I enjoyed working from a family systems perspective, I was firmly entrenched in the cognitive behavioral camp, which was an important distinction in those days. I was trained in behavioral observations and my dissertation capitalized on this methodology. In that work, I demonstrated conclusively that depressed inpatients who were successfully treated with antidepressant medications demonstrated increased extremity movements and social interactions in the lunch room. I even published this work in a prestigious journal (Lyons, Rosen, & Dysken, 1985). The translation of my findings is that when depressed people in the hospital start to get less depressed, they eat (i.e., greater extremity movement) and socialize more (i.e., increased social interaction) during lunch. Although I was excited at the time at how scientific this was, in retrospect, I am underwhelmed. Nobody is going to sit and count arm movements and social exchanges in depressed patients eating to figure out whether or not they are responding to psychotropic medications. Plus, the arm movement in the lunch room was a result of the fact that the patients who were become less depressed were actually more likely to be eating. Not eating is a symptom of depression. There are easier and more direct ways of monitoring this symptom than doing time-sampled behavioral ratings in controlled environments. While molecular measurement is seen as more objective in the logical empiricist tradition, in my experience, the more molecular the measurement process, the more irrelevant it can become to people working in the human service enterprise. The purpose of measurement in human service enterprises is to facilitate the work of these efforts to serve others.

Organization of the Book

The purpose of this book is to provide a conceptual, practical, and scientific framework for a body of ongoing work that I and a large number of colleagues have undertaken in measurement in human service enterprises. The effort is to provide a comprehensive approach to considering measurement as communication. Chapter 2 defines communimetrics and discusses its core principles. Communimetric theory is compared with traditional theories of measurement presently used in human service settings. Chapter 3 describes the process of designing a communimetric measure. The chapter provides practical instruction for those interested in pursuing applications in this approach to measurement. Chapter 4 describes how to evaluate the reliability and validity of a communimetrics; in other words, how you know whether or not you have a "good" communimetric tool. Chapter 5 through 7give detailed examples of three widely used communimetrics measures: the Child and Adolescent Needs and Strengths (CANS), the INTERMED, and the Entrepreneurial League System Assessment (ELSA). Chapter 8 provides a summary and future directions.

Chapter 2
Measurement as Communication

In order to set the stage for understanding communimetrics as a theory of measurement it is important to set the context based on current theories of measurement, of which there are two primary conceptual models—psychometric theories and clinimetric theories. Psychometric theory has two competing approaches within its general framework—classical test theory and item response theory (IRT). The following describes the basic tenets of each of these approaches.

A Brief Review of Current Theories of Measurement

Classical Test Theory

The original psychometric theory is called classical test theory (Nunally, 1976). In this theory, one conceptualizes the universe/population of all possible questions relevant to the measurement of a single construct. Measurement involves the sampling from this population of attributes of the construct and aggregating these sampled attributes to estimate the level of the construct. Picture the population of all possible questions you could ask to measure happiness. Potential questions might involve mood state (e.g., euphoria, blissfulness, sadness) or enjoyment of activities or any number of other aspects of the construct. Classical test theory posits that if you can randomly sample from this population of all possible questions, it is possible to create a valid measure of the construct given a sufficient, representative sample of questions. In order to do a good job of measurement development according to this theory, it is first necessary to define the population of possible items and then adequately sample from it in order to achieve a representative sample. Thus, the usual first step of creating a measure from classical test theory would be to brainstorm as many possible items that might measure some important component of the construct.

Of course it is practically impossible to actually define the population of all possible questions for a construct. Similarly, it is difficult to know a priori whether a particular question actually belongs in the target population or is a better representative

J.S. Lyons, *Communimetrics: A Communication Theory of Measurement in Human Service Settings*,
DOI 10.1007/978-0-387-92822-7_2, © Springer Science+Business Media, LLC 2009

of a different construct. Therefore, classical test theory goes further than just randomly sampling items. It creates a set of statistical strategies that ensure you are sampling items from roughly the same population but not ones that are so overlapping in how people respond to them that they are redundant. Measurement developers using this approach engage in a set of strategies generally referred to as *item analysis* in order to ensure a "Goldilocks" criteria of similar enough, but not too similar, items for all of the items included in a measure.

Item analysis involves the study of the intercorrelations among sets of items and correlations between individual items and total scores. The degree to which items in a set correlate with each other is used as evidence of whether the items are actually measuring the same thing. A correlation of 0.05 between two items suggests they are measuring two different constructs and therefore are not members of the same population. A correlation of 0.95 between two items suggests they are measuring exceptionally overlapping things and are essentially identical from a statistical perspective. A correlation of 0.30 to 0.60 is desirable according to classical test theory (Nunally, 1976). In other words, the items are measuring similar things, but are not too redundant. Negative correlations work the same way. A high negative correlation would be taken as evidence of information redundancy, but in the opposite direction on the construct. Factor analysis can be used to identify the underlying structure of relationships among sampled items. Factor analysis, which is the statistical cornerstone of classical test theory, takes the correlation matrix and places some formal statistical rules on the size of correlations needed to support the claim that the items share a common construct or population (Eysenck, 1971).

Factor analysis as applied to measurement development is essentially an inductive process (putting aside for the moment confirmatory factor analysis). After a set of items are generated it is used to determine statistically whether there is sufficient evidence to suggest that multiple items are measuring the same construct. Many test developers have used the results of factor analyses not only to identify items to include on a test but even to identify and name dimensions of a measure for purposes of scoring and interpretation.

Reliability and validity considerations under classical test theory come directly from the theory behind the choice of items. Although test-retest reliability and inter-rater reliability are important, classical test theory is also used to evaluate measures of transient, subjective states that are neither observable nor necessarily stable. As such, internal consistency reliability has become a commonly used and accepted indicator of reliability. Internal consistency reliability measures the degree to which items of a test correlate with each other—the higher the correlation, the higher the reliability. Generally, the more items that are on a test, the higher the internal consistency reliability will be (Nunally, 1976). Thus, classical test theory, particularly when internal reliability is the only available measure of reliability, implicitly encourages the selection of tests with more items.

Given the care used to measure one construct with multiple items, classical test theory also emphasizes measuring fewer constructs. A good measure, according to this theory, is not multifaceted. Rather, a good measure has a stable factor structure with a discrete, probably low, number of factors. Each of those factors should have discrete validity with other measures of similar (or opposite) constructs. Classical test theory is the measurement foundation behind Eysenck's (1971) classic work on the dimensions of personality and even Leary's (1956) work on the circumplex structure of personality.

Classical test theory generally views *face validity* as the least important of all forms of validity. The most important evidence of validity is captured within the broad area of information that is required to demonstrate *construct validity*. Thus, items do not necessarily have to appear consistent with what they are thought to measure so long as there is statistical evidence that these items really are measuring the construct in question. In fact, for some measures, items that might appear irrelevant can contribute to good measures. There are multiple examples of such items in classically constructed measures, such as the 338 item Minnesota Multiphasic Personality Inventory (MMPI; Butcher, Dahlstrom, Graham, Tellegen, & Kaemmer, 1989). The classic example from the original version of the MMPI was an item involving whether you would sometimes cross the street to avoid running into someone you know. Most people say yes. People who are paranoid as assessed by diagnostic interview are more likely to say no.

In general, classical test theory implicitly defines as reliable and valid longer measures of single (or few) dimensions. Measures with too few items on each dimension or too many dimensions, particularly if they are not orthogonal (i.e., correlated) will be seen as less desirable within this framework. One of the most common reliability criteria in classical test theory is Cronbach's alpha, which is an indicator of the degree to which items on the scale correlate with one another (Cronbach, 1951). The equation for α is:

$$\alpha = \frac{N}{N-1}\left(1 - \frac{\sum_{i=1}^{N} \sigma_{Y_i}^2}{\sigma_X^2}\right)$$

where N is the number of components (items or tests), σ_X^2 is the variance of the observed total test scores, and $\sigma_{y_i}^2$ is the variance of component i.

Cronbach's alpha is biased by the number of items on the scale. The fewer the number of items; the lower the magnitude of the alpha statistic. While corrections exist to this bias (e.g., Allen & Yen, 2002), it remains the case that classical test theory values multiple items to measure single constructs. The history of suspicion of single-item measures rests in classical test theory. Because of the nature of error of measurement, it is certainly true that a linear combination of items is more reliable than an individual item (Nunally, 1976). That, however, does not imply that an individual item cannot be reliable. But you cannot perform an item analysis or factor analysis on a single-item scale, rendering the primary methods of classical test theory useless for these applications. It is in the humanity of scientists to not trust what they cannot study within the range of their methods. If you have a hammer, you tend to look for nails.

Item Response Theory

Item response theory (IRT) approaches the measurement problem in a manner that is quite different from classical test theory. IRT posits the existence of a latent continuum that is the measurable aspect of a particular construct. This continuum can be considered to extend over levels of difficulty. The goal of measurement (at least in human service enterprises) is to reliably and accurately locate a particular person (or perhaps a grouping of people, such as a family) on this continuum relative to all other possible individuals (or comparable groupings). A good measure from this perspective is one that is sensitive across the entire continuum. Therefore, the measure must have the ability to distinguish different people reliably all along the continuum.

The statistical approach to IRT can be quite varied and complex, depending on the number of parameters used to define the continuum. However, in all cases the goal is to identify a set of items that allows for the precise measurement of an individual on the latent continuum or trait. The use of a single parameter model, such as item complexity as used in Rasch scaling (Rasch, 1960/1980), is perhaps the most common approach to measure development and can serve as a constructive example of the implications of IRT for test construction.

In Rasch models, the probability of endorsing an item (if it is discrete) or the population probability of ratings at each level (if it is continuous, such as a Likert scale), is used to define where on the continuum the item is most useful to distinguish respondents (i.e., the separation reliability). The relationship of the item's pattern of difficulty to the rest of the items defines the degree to which the item lies along the latent continuum (i.e., the fit statistic). A good test from a Rasch perspective is one that has items that separate reliability, cover the range of the continuum, and lie along that continuum (Wright & Stone, 1979). Thus, Rasch modeling also consider measures with multiple items on a single dimension to be more reliable and valid. Although there are techniques within IRT that allow you to identify the fewest possible items while maintaining adequate psychometric properties, it remains a significant criterion that the included items cover the latent continuum in terms of varying difficulty (i.e., likelihood of endorsement).

IRT approaches validity from a perspective similar to classical test theory. Statistical relationships between and among items trump other methods for evaluating measures. It is possible that prediction (or statistical criterion) validity is more highly valued in IRT as compared with classical test theory; however, construct validity is again the single most important validity criterion. Face validity is nearly irrelevant as the statistical methods guide the test developer to a greater extent than the perceived experience of the respondent. When items do not fit (the item fit statistic is above 1.6 or so), cognitive testing in which respondents are interviewed while they complete the measure can be used to better understand how people are interpreting the item wording is often recommended.

Clinimetrics

Due to their length and the time and procedural separation between rating, scoring, and interpreting, psychometric measures were not widely accepted in medicine. Although current information technology eliminates many of these challenges, easily accessible, fast computers were not available in the decades in which clinimetrics developed as a theory of measurement. Thus, psychometric tools were seen as burdensome in medical settings. Further, the lack of concern regarding face validity in these approaches sometimes led practicing clinicians to look at the questions and be somewhat skeptical about the measurement process. In an effort to create clinically relevant measurement procedures, physicians and other health researchers have utilized a theoretical approach referred to as clinimetrics (Feinstein, 1987). The stated goal of clinimetrics is to convert "intangible clinical phenomenon into formal specified measurement" (p. 125; Apgar, 1966). Virginia Apgar is generally credited with developing the first measure from this perspective (Apgar). First introduced in 1953, the Apgar is routinely utilized as a health status measure at birth. Clinimetric tools are now quite common in medicine (e.g., Bloem, Beckley, van Hilten, & Roos, 1998; Gates 2000; Hoff, van Hilten, & Roos, 1999; Stone et al., 2001).

Perhaps more than anyone, Feinstein (1999) advocated clinimetrics as a specific theory of measurement. He enumerated six core principles to clinimetrics in comparison with psychometrics:

1. Selection of items is based on clinical rather than statistical criteria.
2. No weighting factors are needed; scoring is simple and readily interpretable.
3. Variables are selected to be heterogeneous rather than homogeneous.
4. The measure must be easy for clinicians to use.
5. Face validity is required.
6. Subjective states are not measured as they are severely limited in terms of source of observation.

Current applications of clinimetrics have some notable limitations (Marx, Bombardier, Hogg-Johnson, & Wright, 2000; Zyzanski & Perloff, 1999). Many clinimetric scales consist of a single item. Attempts to describe complex phenomena with a single item general fail to communicate complexity. For example, a Childhood Global Assessment Scale (Endicott, Spitzer, Fleiss, & Cohen, 1976), which ranges from 0 to 100, can provide a general sense of how the child is doing, but cannot capture individual dimensions of functioning that are useful to clinicians. In addition, single-item measures are not particularly sensitive to change. For these reasons, Zyzanski et al. (1999) and others (e.g., Fava & Belaise, 2005) have called for an integration of clinimetric and psychometric approaches to measurement. Marx, Bombardier, Hogg-Johnson, and Wright (1999) have demonstrated that the two theories can be complementary. Not everyone agrees. Streiner (2003) has gone so far as to argue that clinimetrics is actually a subset of psychometrics, and that for both scientific and communication reasons the word *clinimetric* should be eliminated.

Of course, the distinguishing features described by Feinstein in the process of defining clinimetrics has resulted in most applications involving single items, although in his book Feinstein does not limit clinimetric measures to single items. A single marker of disease severity is the most common type of measure using this framework. Table 2.1 provides an example of a clinimetric measure that is commonly used, the New York Heart Association rating for heart disease. Notice that it assumes the presence of heart disease even at the lowest level. Thus, the concept of normal or normative is either moot or only relevant within the population of people with heart disease.

One of the intriguing characteristics of this measurement approach is that although a key principle of the measurement theory is to keep scoring simple, with no weighting, the actual design of the anchor points creates implicit (and sometimes explicit) weighting of input criteria prior to the clinician's judgment about the rating. Thus, while scoring is simplified, ratings are more complicated. This is how the clinimetric approach differs from psychometrics in the selection of items that reflect clinical judgment. Psychometric theory would emphasize avoiding "double-barreled" items with complex, multiple meanings because they do not tend to scale as well. No such restrictions guide the creation of items in clinimetrics. In fact, if multiple constructs combine to create a continuum of severity, it is desirable to embed all relevant constructs into the anchored definitions of the rating.

The challenge of clinimetric measures is that their use is maximized at the individual patient level, but as you move to higher levels of aggregation, the utility of the measurement approach diminishes. It is hard to monitor and explain transformational processes with clinimetric measures alone. They tend to serve as excellent indicators for defining differences in patient populations but have limited value for outcomes.

Table 2.1 An example clinimetric measure

Class I	Patients with cardiac disease but without resulting limitations of physical activity. Ordinary physical activity does not cause undue fatigue, palpitation, dyspnea, or anginal pain
Class II	Patients with cardiac disease resulting in slight limitations of physical activity. They are comfortable at rest. Ordinary physical activity results in fatigue, palpitation, dyspnea, or anginal pain
Class III	Patients with cardiac disease resulting in marked limitation of physical activity. They are comfortable at rest. Less than ordinary physical activity cases fatigue, palpitation, dyspnea, or anginal pain
Class IV	Patients with cardiac disease resulting in inability to carry on any physical Activity without discomfort. Symptoms of cardiac insufficiency or of the anginal syndrome may be present even at rest. If any physical activity is undertaken, discomfort is increased

The New York Heart Association functional classification.
From The Criteria Committee of the New York Heart Association, Inc. *Diseases of the Heart and Blood Vessels: Nomenclature and Criteria for Diagnosis*. 6th ed. Boston: Little, Brown, 1964.

Comparison of Communimetrics to Psychometrics and Clinimetrics

Measurement can be conceptualized as having at least two distinct phases, input and output. Each aspect requires that decisions be made regarding how that aspect is conceptualized and managed in the measurement process. The input phase involves all the operations of observation and scoring. The input aspects of measurement involve decisions about what to observe, under what conditions to observe, and using what information source for the observation. The output phase involves all the operations involved in using and sharing the measured values. The output process involves decisions about how information is scaled, combined and reported. As demonstrated in Chap. 1 (Fig. 1.2), considering measurement for its communication value shifts the focus from the input side of the measurement process to the output side of the same process. Blanton and Jaccard (2006) have argued that many psychometric measures are arbitrary because the numeric values generated have no grounding in reality. The goal in emphasizing the output applications to the measurement process is to help ensure that the measure is not arbitrary and values generated from a measurement process will be accepted for use within human service enterprises. Therefore, in order to maximize output value, decisions regarding input choices are guided by applications of the measure on the output side.

All measurement theories have to make decisions regarding how the input and output processes interact and inform decisions about each other. Communimetrics differs as a measurement theory from psychometric theories with regard to input, output, and their interaction. Communimetric theory differs from clinimetrics primarily in terms of output decisions.

Input Processes in Measurement

In designing a measure, the first decision that must be made is what aspect of the human condition is to be measured. There are a potentially infinite number of things about people that might be measured; they vary from large, rather global constructs (e.g., job skills, depression) to rather molecular behaviors (e.g., eye blinks, simple arithmetic skills).

The first decision about what construct to measure often has clear and immediate implications as to many of the significant decisions regarding the operations required to measure. For example, if you want to assess eye blink frequency it requires a process that involves prospective, external observation since self-monitoring eye blinking behavior likely influences its frequency. And nobody remembers whether they (or someone else) blinked after even just a short period of time, so recall methods of observation are not feasible. Sadness, on the other hand, is something only available through introspection on the part of the target person.

The second step of the measurement process is in regard to the procedure or operations to be used. With measuring humans, there are three basic choices: self-observation, other observation, and instrument observation. Self-report is preferred when the construct is an internal state that only the individual has access to observe. Knowledge is the best example. The only way one person knows what another person knows is by asking (or testing) them with regard to their knowledge. Other observation is generally used when either self-report is not feasible or cannot be trusted to be accurate. Instrumentation is often seen as the most scientific of all measurement approaches, but it requires a construct for which an observation instrument has been developed. Thus, applications have historically been limited to very specific constructs in which measurement has a clear value and the operation can be automated in some manner (e.g., temperature, weight). Our information culture and the microsizing of computers has created a dramatic increase in instrument measurement in stores and other venues. For example, phenomenon such as Web surfing can be measured using instrumentation (e.g., how many hits on a site). In health care, instrument measurement of humans is widespread, with examples ranging from blood pressure (which still has another observation component in many cases) to positron emission tomography.

The conditions under which a measure is applied is generally the third decision of the measurement input process. In physics and chemistry, there are often powerful assumptions regarding the conditions of measurement (e.g., standard temperature, no gravity). In the measurement of humans, many have tried to be equally rigorous, but the realities of the processes necessary to obtain information often compromise rigid rules regarding the conditions of measurement. Standardized tests in the education field are good examples of attempts to enforce routine conditions on the measurement process. People administering standardized tests have a set of rules and time frames that they must follow in order to ensure comparability in conditions across different measurements. The administration of these standard educational tests via computer has made this type of procedural control more efficient. Other examples include measurement at intake into a clinic or program followed by repeated readministration of the measure at fixed intervals (e.g., every 3 months, at discharge).

The final consideration, although not necessarily the last, in the input process of measurement is the satisfaction of whomever must complete the measure regarding its ease of use, suitability, etc. These characteristics are included what has been called “face validity,” i.e., the measure is valid on the face of it. Existing measurement theories weigh the importance of this consideration differentially.

The Output Process in Measurement

There are also a number of important decisions that the developer of a measure must confront regarding the output of the measurement process. Scaling is the first decision of the output process. What is the unit of measure? How many levels exist in each item? What is the proposed relationship among those levels? Historically, scaling has been categorized as categorical, ordinal, interval, and ratio. Categorical scales describe things in discrete groups that have no hierarchy. Ordinal scales have a hierarchy, but the differences among levels in this hierarchy are not comparable. Interval scales order levels in a fashion that allows for an assumption of equal differences among levels. Ratio scales have an absolute zero. Ratio scales are thought to be rare for constructs of interest within human service enterprises.

Within these standard categorizations of scales, there is further differentiation. For example, Gutman scales are a form of an ordinal scale in which each new response, when endorsed, requires that all previous responses have been endorsed as well. The classic example of a Gutman scale measures racial discrimination using something like the following questions:

1. Would you be OK with a person of [insert race] living in your town or city?
2. Would you be OK with a person of [insert race] living in your neighborhood?
3. Would you be OK with a person of [insert race] living on your street?
4. Would you be OK with a person of [insert race] living next door to you?
5. Would you be OK with a person of [insert race] living in your house?

If you said yes to question 4, then you would obviously have said yes to questions 1 through 3, but may not necessarily had said yes to item 5.

There are other types of ordinal scales: frequencies, class rank, power rankings of sports teams, etc. are all ordinal in their scaling properties. These scales are easy to use and understand, but are limited in statistical applications as they are less easily combined, and often you can't use parametric statistics with them. Frequency scales (i.e., raw counts) are often mistakenly thought of as interval scales.

Within interval scales, the most common type is the Likert Scale (Anastasi, 1968; Nunally, 1976). Generally, Likert scales assess either agreement or intensity, which is sometimes used to convert frequency measurement into an interval scale.

Agree completely	Never
Agree somewhat	Rarely
Neither agree or disagree	Sometimes
Disagree somewhat	Often
Disagree completely	Always

There are other types of ratings besides Likert Scales, such as visual analogs and 0 to 100 ratings, which are thought to normally function as interval scales. By and large, it is accepted while these types of scales can be assumed to function as interval scales; however, it is a good idea to test any scale as it functions to ensure this important characteristic.

Once scaling decisions have been made, the next decision about measurement output is how to combine items. It is on this decision that the various measurement theories diverge most dramatically, so this topic is discussed in greater detail within each of the major theories. However, overall, decisions have to be made about which items can be added together and in what fashion in order to create scores that are used as the primary outputs of the measurement process. With psychometric theories, single items are thought to not make reliable measures; therefore, some combination is always required. With clinimetric and communimetric measures, single items can make reliable measures, so the decision making in this regard is different. Generally, with clinimetrics only single-item scales are used, so decisions about combinations are moot.

As discussed, Blanton and Jaccard (2006) have described the problem of arbitrary metrics in psychological measures. These authors define arbitrary as "when it is not known where a given score locates an individual on the underlying psychological dimension or how a one-unit change on the observed score reflects the magnitude of change on the underlying dimension" (p. 28). In other words, scores on many measures do not have independent relationships with the degree (e.g., severity, difficulty, intensity) of the construct purported to be measures: A 15 on the Beck Depression Inventory is not tied directly to a degree of depression itself. These authors press for tying levels of measures to real-world, meaningful events as necessary to making measures reliable, valid, and not arbitrary.

The third decision about output processes in measurement is how the scores are presented, displayed, or otherwise communicated. Some measures use normative transformations, such as T scores (mean of 50 with standard deviation of 10). Other measures use total scores or profiles of scores. Some strategy is necessary to ensure that the scores have meaning to those who intend to use them or that individuals who utilize the scores can be educated to interpret them appropriately. Psychometric measures must develop some strategy to ensure meaningfulness. Both clinimetric and communimetric measures are designed for immediate meaning, at least at the level of a single item.

The final characteristic of the output process is whether the use of the measure has any impact on the people who receive the information. That is, does the information taken from the measure within the human services setting actually result in a change of behavior or performance. Although a validity consideration for all approaches to measurement, this measure utility or impact is not a primary consideration in the design of measures developed out of psychometric theories. This is a central output consideration for communimetric measures.

The Relationship of Input and Output Process

In the measurement development process, depending on the theory, complex relationships exist between input and output processes. In particular, in psychometric theories results of statistical analysis of item performance from the output processes have direct implications for the design of input processes. Both classical test theory and IRT have specific, well-defined characteristics for a well functioning item. Those characteristics involve the statistical performance of the item relative to other items, and sometimes, an external criterion. An item that does not perform statistically in a manner consistent with the theory, then it should be removed from the input process. Thus, measurement development is generally defined by findings from the input side of the measurement process. For example, in classical test theory there is an optimal correlation among items and between an item and the total scale. Two items that have a high correlation are considered redundant from an information perspective and one is generally removed. An item with too low of a correlation to the total score is thought to be measuring a different construct and therefore, it is eliminated. If a subset of items can predict the total score of a larger set of items, then a shorter version of the measure (i.e., the subset) is recommended.

Item-response theory uses item fit statistics to determine whether the item is performing as expected. In other words, is the probably of endorsing different levels of an item (i.e., termed item difficulty in Rasch modeling) consistent with that item residing on the underlying continuum shared by other items in the sample. In addition, item-response theory looks for items that spread across likelihood of endorsement (i.e., item difficulty) to ensure that items are included that are sensitive at different levels of the construct. Failure on these input analyses leads to changes in the input process. Thus, if too many items are "easy" (i.e., frequently endorsed), it will result in an insensitive measure across the latent trait and the measure will have a ceiling effect. More difficult items must be identified. Similarly, if there are two many "difficult" items (i.e., rarely endorsed), then the measure has a floor effect and easier items must be added. A shorter version from an IRT is a scale that has a uniform distribution of items across levels of difficulty while maintaining good item fit statistics on the continuum.

Input and Output Processes in Human Service Enterprises

Human service enterprise settings have very different priorities than research settings. Accommodating these technical and contextual requirements requires a broad scope for models of measurement. The measurement model must include guidelines for utility in operations as well as reliability and validity. It is not necessarily true (as psychometric measurement theory assumes) that if you develop a good measure from an item analysis, it will result in a useful measure within a human service enterprise. Measures intended for the assessment of transformational offerings should be easy to use and brief. Their output should be clear, unambiguous, relevant, easy to translate into intervention planning recommendations, and accessible to providers, consumers, and policy makers. Classical test theory, IRT, and clinimetrics are not able to fully inform the development of measures meeting these requirements in human service enterprise applications.

As discussed in Chap. 1, in entities that provide help for people, the primary role of measurement is to communicate. That communication is first between the consumer and the provider (e.g., what do we need to work on together?), but the communication can be far more complex than that. Often, human services are paid for by the government or other entities. Thus, third parties (the consumer is the first and the provider is the second party in the transaction) are involved in payment for these interventions. Communication between providers and payor also is important. In addition, fourth parties are involved, including accreditation and other entities that monitor human service enterprises. In some situations, even fifth, sixth, and seventh parties are involved because the nature of the intervention requires the participation of multiple system partners. For example, in the child-serving system, it is not unheard of that child welfare, juvenile justice, mental health, and educational representatives are involved with the same youth. Communication with each of these parties is important to the work. That communication should focus on the nature of the work—the *human* in the human service enterprise. Measurement as communication is different in some important ways than other forms of measurement.

Principles of Communimetrics

Considering the communication value of a measure from the beginning changes some core principles of measurement design. This is particularly true when a constitutive view of communication is taken in which communication is viewed as the creation of a shared meaning. There are six key principles of measurement as communication—communimetrics:

1. Each item has implications for differential action.
2. Levels of each item are immediately translatable into action.
3. Measurement must remove the context, including:
   a. Services already in place
   b. Culture
   c. Development
4. Measurement is descriptive and minimizes cause–effect assumptions.
5. Observation windows can be trumped by the action levels.
6. Information integration

Each Item Has Implications for Differential Action

Like clinimetric measures, communimetric tools are designed so that they can operate at the item level. As described, clinimetric measures have proved false the psychometric theory position that only multiple item scales are reliable by demonstrating the feasibility and utility of single-item scales in medical settings. Communimetrics also emphasizes the use of single items, but also encourages multiple item approaches to allow comprehensive assessments of multiple constructs to facilitate decision making and outcome monitoring.

Given the action orientation of communimetric tools, items are included in a measure if they have a potentially meaningful relationship to what happens next in the human service enterprise. In other words, the assessment is a planning process for any interventions that follows; items exist to inform choices among possible interventions or approaches. An item that is irrelevant to the planning process should not be included.

Levels of Items Translate Immediately to Action

A unique requirement of a communimetric measure is that the levels of measurement on each item should translate into action. In other words, the individual items are selected to guide decision making. The levels of these items should further guide decision making by indicating what level of service effort is required. A standard four-point communimetric scale might look like the following:

0 No evidence, no need for action
1 Watching waiting/prevention or keeping an eye on something
2 Action is needed
3 Immediate or intensive action is needed

Thus the design of the levels of an item on which ratings are made should immediately communicate the meaning of the item from a planning perspective. Here would be an example of a communimetric scale for a strategic planning process:

0 Not relevant
1 Parking lot
2 Issue to be addressed
3 Priority issue

An issue that is classified as not relevant can be dropped from the discussion. A "parking lot" issue is something that isn't immediately important, but should be returned to at a more appropriate time. Items rated a 2 or 3 should be addressed in the strategic plan with those being rated a 3 taking priority.

Strength-based planning has increasingly become a best practice in child serving systems (Healy, 2005). The following is an example of a communimetric scale from the Child and Adolescent Needs and Strengths for strengths measurement:

0 Centerpiece strength
1 Useful strengths
2 Identified strength
3 No strengths identified

In this model, a centerpiece strength can be used as the focus of a strength-based plan. For example, if a child is removed from his or her parents due to abuse or neglect, but grandparents are available who are willing to take the child into their home, that is a centerpiece family strength. A useful strength is something that can be included in a strength-based plan but cannot serve as a centerpiece (e.g., knitting when stressed, enjoying singing in a choir, youth soccer for an 8 year old). An identified strength gives you a window into where a strength could be built (e.g., a particular vocational interest in the absence of any knowledge or skills), and if no strength is identified that would preclude its inclusion in a strength-based plan. Thus, using this communimetric strength scale, strengths rated a 0 or 1 could be included in strength-based planning and those rated 2 or 3 might become the focus of strength identification and building efforts.

The action orientation of a communimetric tool is one of its greatest strengths. It eliminates the arbitrariness of a Likert scale as there is a clear link between the level of the measure and the external world. It makes the link between assessment and intervention planning transparent in support of supervision and other forms of accountability. It facilitates a full understanding of when interventions are no longer necessary, although meaningful applications for outcomes management. The levels of the items communicate between assessor and various parties who might be involved in providing transformational experiences based on the assessment findings. People who are assessed often report that this is the aspect that they most appreciate because it provides them with a framework for the work they have ahead of them if they wish to change aspects of their lives. However, the action orientation is not without controversy.

By establishing a clear, visible link between assessment processes and interventions opportunities for accountability are dramatically enhanced. I was doing training in Florida on a mental health version of the CANS and I presented the basic action levels: no evidence, watchful waiting/prevention, action, and immediate/intensive action. Someone came up to me at the break and said, "Well John, you realize this means we have to do something." They were quite distressed at thinking that once the tool had been applied it became clear to youth and families that something had to be done. I was struck by the irony of this concern. I answered, "That's exactly what it means. If you rate an item 2 or 3, then something has to be done." Isn't that the point of assessment after all—to figure out what needs to be addressed?

In New Jersey, I completed training and e-mailed people who had passed and not passed the certification test demonstrating reliability. One particular person was not reliable, and I e-mailed her with the news and feedback on what she missed. Essentially she had consistently underestimated needs of the youth in the test vignette. Reacting to this feedback, she replied that underestimating needs was just how they worked at her office. She stated that they really didn't have any options available to serve children and youth and had just found that they were better off pretending that treatment needs just didn't exist. Of course, this is missing the point of the framework for these types of tools. It isn't about pretending everything is OK. The process should be about identifying needs and if you can't meet them, then you have succeeded in identifying an unmet need. Documenting unmet (or unmeetable) needs becomes important information for improving the human service enterprise in the future.

This concern about action continues to be a sticking point for some people as they attempt to implement communimetric tools in human service enterprises. But just because you identify an item that requires action, it does not mean that a specific action should automatically follow. Because of the fifth principle of communimetric measurement, "It is about the what, not the why," there is no need to define precisely what must be done. In fact, creating hypotheses about the why (i.e., cause-and-effect relationship leading to the identified need), is the nature of transformational interventions. It is one thing to identify whether an entrepreneur has human resource management skills; it is a different thing to figure out how to help that specific person develop his or her skills. Or, it is one thing to say that a child or youth is misbehaving at school, it is a different process to determine why. The specific intervention is based on a hypothesis of the why. In the communimetric measurement model, assessment is describing the target of the intervention. The choice of interventions is often based on a hypothesis about a potential cause of the target.

An additional concern that is sometimes raised about action levels is that they are somehow circular. In other words, by defining the ratings based on actions to follow, the assessment is no longer independent of these actions. I would argue that it is true that the ratings are not independent, but that this interdependence is a good thing and not a problem within the context of the human service enterprise. Here is where the business context is different than a scientific perspective that might require that any measurement is independent of all others. It is quite valuable to understand how assessors are conceptualizing needs and strengths from the perspective of the enterprise. The action levels make this possible. A constitutive form of communication in which meaning is made among parties in the transaction through a consensus on the relationship of the level of need to the level of intervention is a major benefit of this approach.

Considering Context

A second unique feature of a communimetric approach is that the person(s) completing the measure is required to consider the larger context in which the measurement is occurring to prevent undue influence of contextual factors on the description of the person or entity under consideration. This characteristic is radically different than traditional scientific measurement, which attempts to control contextual factors methodologically rather than conceptually. Physics measures in a vacuum. Chemistry measures at a set temperature and barometric pressure. Such methodological control is not possible in human service settings. The following are some contextual considerations that might influence the process of establishing action levels.

Services in Place

The purpose of measurement in service delivery is to determine what actions must be taken. If actions are already being taken, that changes the context of the measurement process. That is, you are measuring things that are the targets of the enterprise.

If you are providing business incubation you are measuring factors related to entrepreneurial success. If you are providing health care, you are measuring things related to health status, level of functioning and well-being. If you are providing vocational services, you are measuring things related to job readiness.

If you are in the middle of providing interventions in support of improving targets of the enterprise, then it falls to reason that you would expect change in these targets as an outcome of these activities. That's what transformative offerings are all about. However, many such interventions may work only while they are active. For example, a person may perform adequately at work only when a job coach is present. Remove the job coach and performance deteriorates. Or, a person with a severe mental illness may only be symptom free when they take medication as prescribed. The intervention meets the need, but does not resolve it.

In order to understand the need for ongoing interventions, those that must remain in place to secure success are different from those interventions that have accomplished their objectives and can be ended. Traditional measurement approaches do not make this distinction. They describe the status of the person *regardless* of the service context. A person performing well at work with a job coach is no different than a person performing well with one. A person who is not symptomatic on medication is no different from the person who no longer needs to take his or her medication at all. In traditional measurement, interpretation of the meaning of the measure requires one to consider the service context after the measurement has been completed, as part of the analytic work. This ad hoc interpretation of contextual factors creates all sorts of problems with communication.

Consider the following example. Residential treatment is a common intervention for children and adolescents with severe or complex needs. This form of treatment involves placing the youth into a therapeutic living situation where he or she might stay for treatment from 30 days to several years. The treatment often works and youth get better during the episode of care. The youth then is returned to home or back to the community in a foster home or perhaps even an independent living environment. I have often heard it reported that parents and community providers experience the reported status of children and youth using standard measures as misleading, saying something to the effect of, "The residential provider says that the youth was doing fine, but as soon as they got back home everything began to fall apart again." This miscommunication occurs because the residential provider is describing how the child is doing *in their setting*, which has all sorts of therapeutic components and behavioral controls.

A communimetric measure requires that the communicator represent the child or youth's status independent of the service setting. So instead of describing how the youth is doing in residential treatment, the communicator is instructed to assess how that individual would be expected to function without all the supports inherent in the residential treatment center. Thus, in order to effectively communicate using a structured measure, the residential rater has to distinguish setting effects (improvements that come from living in a structured setting) vs. treatment effects (improvements that transcend the structure setting that will generalize to other environments).

Culture

Over the past several decades, social scientists and service delivery systems have become sensitized to the complexity of addressing cultural issues effectively in practice. There is overwhelming evidence that racial and ethnic disparities exist in many human service systems in the United States (e.g., Smedly, Stith, & Nelson, 2003). Addressing cultural issues is complex, however. There are actually three different strategies that are necessary to effectively address cultural issues in human service enterprises.

Treating Different People Differently

The primary focus of cultural-based initiatives in service delivery has been an effort to teach service delivery systems to treat different people differently. This skill set is often referred to as cultural sensitivity. Some people use the term *cultural competence*, but I would argue that this term is an oxymoron. The opposite of competence is incompetence, and anyone who goes around referring to others as "incompetent" is likely not sensitive to others. Thus, it seems preferable to choose to use the term *cultural sensitivity* to describe the skill of adjusting the human service enterprises to account for relevant variations in culture.

An obvious example of cultural sensitivity comes from mental health. If a person is an active member of a Pentecostal church, he or she may talk in tongues during religious services. This behavior does not make the person psychotic. The same vocalization patterns exhibited by someone walking down the street or being interviewed in an emergency department might be seen as compelling evidence of a symptom of psychosis.

I recently received an e-mail from a colleague about a case of a young woman in Oregon. Her grandfather had died and she had been close to him. He was the *pater familia* and a source of significant support for this adolescent girl. Following his death, she reported talking to her grandfather and her psychiatrist diagnosed her as psychotic and sought to start her on antipsychotic medication due to the presence of delusional thinking. Here's the problem with this situation. The young lady was Native American. In her culture, speaking to dead ancestors is a traditional way of describing the continuing influence of a lost loved one, just like a religious person may refer to speaking to God.

Traditional measurement approaches try to measure completely independent of cultural influences. So ratings assessing delusions or hallucinations might be defined in a way that a Native American or devoted religious person might respond to in the affirmative. This approach forces cultural sensitivity to occur after the measurement process is complete as a part of interpreting the numbers. While measuring independently from cultural influences is reasonable, and perhaps even optimal, for scientific investigation, it places enormous challenges on information collected in service delivery settings. Without detailed knowledge about the cultures of individuals involved in transactions, it is exceptionally difficult to recreate potential influences with aggregated data. Thus, it is difficult to know whether disparities exist in assessment or interventions.

Some psychometric measures, such as the Cardiff Anomalous Perception Scale (Bell, Halligan, & Ellis, 2006) address this issue by making all items ipsative; that is, based on the individual's open experience set, e.g., "Do you ever think that food or drink tastes much stronger than it normally would?" This represents a reasonable alternative to considering cultural factors prior to establishing the level of an item. In this model, you allow the individual to correct for cultural influences prior to answering the questions. However, such instructions are never a part of psychometric measurement.

In the traditional model cultural factors become variables that you have to control in order to interpret information. Large sample sizes and/or sophisticated multivariate statistical techniques are required to ensure that standards of cultural sensitivity are met. You can't really even report the frequency with which people report "delusional thinking" without first factoring in the degree to which some cultural factors might influence this rate. Placing this level of interpretative responsibility at the analytical level (following scoring) is inconsistent with effective communication because the raw data collected might be misleading unless specific analytical procedures are first applied. At the individual person level, the implications are more complicated and you are left trying to decide whether or not the information is meaningful. A clearly interpretable rating that does not require scoring is the clearest form of communication.

The traditional alternative to understanding contextual variables analytically is to create different measures for different contexts. This is one of many reasons why so many different measures exist in the human service enterprise. However, the use of culturally specific measurement is limited if you want to be able to draw conclusions about human service enterprises in cross-cultural settings or if you ever want to understand the role of culture in the functioning of these enterprises.

Communimetric measures build the concept of cultural sensitivity directly into the measurement process. Before an action level is determined, culture must be considered. If something is a behavioral norm in an individual's culture, then it is not a need. Family involvement manifests itself in very different ways across ethnic and cultural groups. Consideration of these factors must occur before one could identify actionable family needs or strengths.

An exception to this rule exists when a specific culture has a behavioral norm that is outside the range of nonculture-based behavioral norms. Behaviors such as corporal punishment and female castration are examples of these types of behaviors; normative in some cultures, but widely unacceptable across cultures. For example, a parent beating his or her child would be described as physical abuse in the United States, Canada, and Europe regardless of the culture of the person for which that behavior is described.

Treating Different People the Same

Cultural sensitivity does not apply to all situations. There are situations in which we must learn to treat different people the same regardless of their cultural differences. Racial disparities in health care and employment are important examples of these problems. For example, there is substantial evidence that in the United States, African Americans are more likely to be admitted to the hospital and receive lower-quality outpatient treatment than do Caucasians (Smedly et al., 2003). Nobody believes that race should explain the utilization of health care or employment rates and income levels. If a measurement process is to be useful from a cultural perspective in a delivery system, it should be able to be used to identify and address disparities.

Addressing Cultural Needs

The third way in which culture should be addressed within a delivery system is that sometimes specific culture-based needs can be identified. Once identified, the system should be able to address them. Language is an obvious one. If a person of a family member does not speak the primary language in a jurisdiction, then he or she needs help to ensure that effective communication can be accomplished. Without everyone in the process having a full voice, it is impossible to have a fully effective system. Other cultural needs might include access to rituals (e.g., food, holidays, music) or cultural identity and/or stress. Often, families that emigrate to the United States experience complex intergenerational stress in that the children in the family are sometimes more readily affected by U.S. cultural influences, creating tensions with parents.

Development

A third contextual factor can be development. We have dramatically different expectations with regard to behavior and performance based on age, both chronological and developmental. All 3 year olds have anger control problems, so this is irrelevant to any assessment of behavioral health. A 15 year old or a 30 year old who has the anger control skills of a 3 year old would represent a problem, however. We don't expect an infant to be able to toilet himself or herself. By around 2 years old, this becomes a societal expectation, and the failure of an older child to successful toilet himself or herself is considered an actionable need.

Recreation functioning requires entirely different considerations based on age and development. Children do not engage in the same recreational activities as adolescents. Young adults do not engage in the same recreational activities as older adults. If you want to understand recreational functioning in terms of the need for interventions, it is essential to do it within a developmentally appropriate framework.

Measurement is Descriptive

In the context of measurement in human services, causal relationships are complex and judgments with regard to cause-and-effect is subject to substantial error. For instance, in behavioral health, there is no known pathogen. Therefore, jumping to a cause of any symptom or behavior is likely to be wrong. So, at least for the majority of items, communimetric tools tend to focus on describing actionable conditions rather than interpreting them within a causal framework.

In trainings, I often use the mantra, "It is about the what, not about the why." In my experience this aspect of the communimetric measurement facilitates its use in constitutive communication. In many situations within human service enterprises, shame and blame come from the why. Stigma comes from the why. When you focus on the what—the description of what the needs are without initially trying to determine the cause of these needs—it serves as an engagement strategy. The fact that you are homeless is one thing. The reasons you are homeless are a different conversation.

Treatment interventions are almost invariably directed to the theory of why. So the nature of the intervention requires a hypothesis about the why to go along with the description provided in the assessment. This relationship between assessment and treatment allows you to use communimetric tools to pursue person-driven planning. In other words, the assessment process is used to reach a consensus about what is going on (i.e., constitutive communication). The individual or family generates hypotheses as to why these things are happening; then the professional brings in evidence-based approaches to address this proposed cause. If the first intervention doesn't work, then a new hypothesis is generated.

Use of Time Frames (Windows of Observation)

All measures require a definition of the time frame over which an observation can occur. As a thinking tool, communimetrics has a different philosophy in this regard. Time windows for observations (e.g., 30 days, 24 hours, etc) are recommended, but they exist to remind people using these tools that ratings should be fresh; however, these ratings must be implemented with flexibility. At the end of the day, the role of a measurement process in the human services context in which communimetric tools are used is to establish actionable items. Thus, the action levels take precedence over the time frames. Time frames are only relevant as they inform action levels.

For example, in the Child and Adolescent Needs and Strengths (CANS, see Chap. 5), a 30-day time frame is used unless an item specifies otherwise. However, a rater can change his or her rating based on the specific situation. My favorite example of this procedure is an example of doing an assessment with a young adult who is in the hospital after a car accident. Let's say for sake of illustration that the young man drank, drove, and crashed his car. As a result of the crash, he ended up hospitalized in a coma for 90 days. If you were charged with planning his treatment post-discharge from the hospital, would you argue that he has been "clean and sober" for 90 days? Of course not. He's been in a coma. In fact, his substance use need would probably best be described knowing how he was doing prior to his accident, not during his hospital stay.

Information Integration

Communimetric measurement is an information integration strategy. Information integration refers to the process whereby multiple inputs are combined to generate a measurement. Therefore, communimetrics operates at a higher level of measurement than the direct application of instrumentation. A lab assay applies measurement processes to biological materials. A ruler applies its metric to an observed distance. The direct application of instrumentation to generate measurement is the foundation of science. However, when information is used in human service settings, it is often necessary to measure at what might be called the level of *executive function*. This type of measurement process requires the combination of multiple and potentially competing measurements or observations into a single measure. Psychometrics accomplishes information integration by asking multiple questions to the same source to measure a specific construct. That requirement can be limiting. For example, if a clinician is attempting to measure depression, self-reported symptoms are one input; however, observed mood, physical activity levels, and reports from significant others, are all relevant to that measurement process. The clinical judgment of whether or not depression is evident and to what degree is based on the integration of measurement from multiple sources. Any clinician will tell you that single-source measurement is inherently limited across a cohort of assessments.

In children's mental health, the Child Behavioral Checklist (CBCL; Achenbach, 1991) has versions for parents, teachers, therapists, and youth. The correlations among these versions are generally quite low. Accordingly, these findings demonstrate that working independently, different people describe the same youth differently. However, at some point everyone should come to agreement about what the youth needs and what should be done about it. The disagreement among the multiple sources only prepares you for how much work you will have to do to reach consensus. The consensus is necessary to actually intervene.

Similarly, if a business incubator is attempting to understand a start-up company's market potential, the inputs into that assessment are also multiple. It may include the novelty of the product, its cost, the existence of a known market, and so forth. Each of these factors, all relevant to market potential, require different measurement processes. However, the venture capitalist still must put all of those inputs together to make his or her judgment with regard to a new business's market potential.

Team Decision Making and Strategic Planning

Communimetrics is designed to operate at the level of the person overseeing the implementation of the interventions within a human service enterprise, e.g., the clinician or the venture capitalist. In fact, the design of the communimetric approach is uniquely suited for team decision-making measurement. Any strategic planning process can be conceptualized as measurement: What do we have? What do we need? What should be done to move forward? These are all higher-order measurements. Teams convene to provide multiple inputs into these planning processes. The contribution of each team member can be conceptualized as a measurement input, and the output of the team similarly can be seen as a measurement. Communimetric measures function well as outputs of team measurement processes. Again, the team is generally engaged in constitutive communication, creating meaning.

Self-Report and Communimetrics

Measurement strategies that have the respondent directly answer questions on a survey are commonly called *self-report*. In many ways, self-report measurement is a field in and of itself, as the nuances of how you obtain accurate and useful information directly from target respondents has received much investigation. Self-report methods of measurement have a number of important advantages:

- They are direct. The target person is the one who responds to the questions or item prompts. There is no interpretive filter by an observing other.
- They provide a certain level of confidentiality; sometimes the illusion is even greater confidentiality than is actually the case.
- They are inexpensive. Generally the target person is not paid to complete the measure, so from the human service enterprise perspective, it is provided at almost no cost.

Getting information directly from the individuals you are seeking to measure makes a great deal of sense. Who knows you better than yourself? As long as the information sought is open to self-observation, then in theory at least, it is accessible to self-report measurement. And, things that are never available to observation (e.g., a feeling state, self-esteem) are only accessible via some form of self-report.

There is a body of research that suggests people are often more comfortable telling secrets to a computer administered survey than to a person-administered approach (Lyons, Howard, O'Mahoney, & Lish, 1997). This suggests that there is something about interacting with a form that is different than interacting with a person. The relational aspects of the presence of the other person might influence how we choose to present ourselves. Relationships can influence differential responses depending on the method of inquiry. This effect appears despite the reality that eventually other people will view the person's responses to the survey questions even if they were provided only to a computer. Consequently, some form of faux confidentiality effect appears to be operating. Perhaps if you don't have to witness the other person's reaction to your responses, you don't worry about those reactions as much as if the other person is sitting with you and you can directly observe her or him as you answer questions.

Once you consider self-report from a communication perspective, it shifts how you think about self-report methods and may lead you to consider whether it really is a separate method at least in human service enterprise applications. Table 2.2 inventories three basic approaches to self-report. Instructions only is the type of measurement process in which you simply give the respondent the survey, with instructions written on the survey, and ask him or her to complete it independently. With support involves working with the respondent to make sure he or she understands the instructions and what each question is attempting to measure. Collaboration means that the respondent and a professional sit down together and talk through the survey so that the respondent can fill it out. Which strategy you choose will depend on a variety of factors, including the difficulty of the construct measured and the age, developmental stage, and reading level of the respondent.

Table 2.2 also contains three basic methods for interview. Open-ended interviews are simply discussions. They have no required structure. Semistructured interviews provide some basic structural guidelines in terms of topics and general questions, but limit the structure to more global topics than specific questions. Structured interviews, on the other had, are fully elaborated. Questions are provided to the interviewer, who is expected to ask them verbatim, and the respondent is given closed-ended response options and asked to endorse one (or more) for each question.

If you consider the options in Table 2.2, you will see there is hardly any difference between a collaborative model of self-report and the structured interview technique. The difference may be only who wields the pencil (or access to the keypad) to actually answer the questions. In self-report, the respondent generally completes the form, while in a structured interview the interviewer does.

One could actually make a similar interpretation of the other pairs of methods. In some ways (although not all), self-report with support and semistructured interviews are similar in that they both give a bit more leeway for the person completing the form to interpret the information herself or himself without the input of others. And, only self-report and open-ended interviews both give the person completing the form a great deal of freedom to interpret the measure in any fashion. The only difference is in the range of response options. Generally, an interview has more

Table 2.2 Basic Methodological Approaches to Collecting Self-Report and Interview Information

Self-report
Instructions only. Informant is given form and completes it independently
Support. Informant completes form but is allowed to ask questions and seek assistance as needed
Collaboration. The form is completed as the informant works through the questions with someone to read and clarify the questions and possible responses.
Interview
Open-ended. Interviewer asks general questions and allows informant to determine the direction of the interview
Semistructured. Interviewer as a set of defined questions but allows the informant to deviate somewhat based on the content of the interview
Structured. Interview follows strict order of questions and requests that the informant answer the questions in order

response options than a self-report questionnaire (although this is not an absolute requirement).

Exploring Myths in Measurement

Merriam-Webster defines a myth as "(a) a popular belief or tradition that has grown up around something or someone; (**b**) an unfounded or false notion." Based on research using psychometric theories and research samples, there are some myths that have become accepted truths of measurement. Primary among these beliefs are the following notions:

- Add or subtract an item from a scale and you change the reliability and validity.
- Change the order of the items and you change the reliability and validity.
- Single-item scales are not likely to be reliable or valid.
- All measures must be "normed."

As may be obvious from the prior description of measurement of communimetrics, this theory of measurement questions these four beliefs. Since these ideas come close to reaching the perceived level of "truth" in the field of measurement, it is worth discussing why a communimetrics perspective does not accept the truth of these assertions.

Item Inclusion and Sequence

In order to understand these first two beliefs, it is important to consider the context of most measurement research in social sciences. The vast majority of measurement research is accomplished by psychologists in university settings. These researchers balance their need to both teach and engage in productive research by establishing subject pools, often through introductory classes. For example, most introduction to psychology classes provider a very low-grade Sophie's Choice—either write a paper or participate in a research study. Not surprising, most students choose the research participation over writing an additional paper. Often psychologists are sometimes seen as tricky or manipulative in their research, so these naïve subjects are likely wondering what the purpose of the study in which they are participating. In this context, of course, the inclusion or exclusion of an item makes a difference, or the order of the items shifts how subjects might respond to different questions. They are likely attempting to guess what the experimenter is looking for and tailoring their communication consistent with an emerging (and possibly shifting) theory. This logic does not apply to people seeking assistance in the human service enterprise.

Although there are a large number of studies exploring these issues, they share the same basic method: the study of college undergraduates. As an example, Dahlstrom,

Brooks, and Peterson (1990) demonstrate that scrambling items on the Beck Depression Inventory results in a higher estimated level of depression than does ordering them by severity (as is the standard approach with this measure). Of course the subjects for this study were undergraduate women at the University of North Carolina at Chapel Hill, not people seeking treatment for their depression. Knowles 1988 with a sample of 120 undergraduate psychology and human development students at the University of Wisconsin at Green Bay demonstrated that the later an item occurred in a sequence, the higher its correlation with the total score. This finding was used to posit that over the course of the experiment, the subject was becoming increasingly self-aware (i.e., activated self-schema), and thus the subject is more accurate and reliable over time.

However, there is evidence even with college samples in support of the communimetric perspective. Hamilton and Shuminsky 1990 followed the Knowles study to demonstrate that contextual differences can influence the importance of the serial position of an item. In their study of 242 college undergraduates at the University of Colorado at Colorado Springs, these researchers use Fenigstein and Levine's 1984 story writing method to induce either an internal (self-awareness) or external focus. The subjects participating in the internal focus group were not affected by the serial position of items. Subjects in the external focus group replicated the findings of Knowles (1988).

It is an easy argument that people seeking help from the human service enterprise would be far more likely to be self-aware regarding the reasons that they are seeking help than your average college undergraduate participating in a study that is not necessarily relevant to them other than helping them avoid writing a paper. In fact, I would argue that often self-awareness of need is what actually brings an individual in contact with the human service enterprise in the first place. While this is not always true (e.g., court-mandated treatment for mental health or substance abuse), it is generally true. Regardless, people are coming to human service enterprises for help. These individuals are fundamentally different from college freshman participating in an experiment. There are very few people who would argue that the best way to get accurate information from people in need is to force them to answer a standard set of questions in a standard format. Reliability and validity of a measure are just technical aspects of accuracy. Most experienced human service providers learn that they need to let people tell their stories to start—however they tell it. This builds the type of relation that is required to get accurate information. So in fact, a standard battery of questions that may or may not be relevant to the person seeking assistance is potentially off-putting.

Individual Items

The potential reliability of single items has been demonstrated multiple times in the field of medicine. From the Apgar forward, most clinimetric measures are single items that result in reliable and valid information. Therefore, this myth does not reflect the existing literature. That being said, it remains the case that linear combinations of variables are generally more reliable than single variables (within that set). But it is a non sequitur to argue that a linear combination of relatively unreliable items is more reliable and, therefore, valid than a well-constructed single item. Anderson et al. (2003) demonstrated that item reliability can be obtained prospectively and with chart audit across a range of 45 different items of a communimetric tool.

Norms

Creating norms for various measures has been a tradition within psychometrics for a long time. The primary purpose of a norm is to try to give meaning to an otherwise arbitrary metric. By creating a standard scale with an identified and known mean and standard deviation it is possible to create clear expectations about the placement of an individual relative to all other individuals in the distribution of scores from that measure. We know that an IQ of 100 is perfectly normal (i.e., average) because 100 is the defined mean of the normative IQ score. Further, we know that an IQ of 130 is two standard deviations above the mean, indicating that 2.5% of the population has IQ scores at this level or higher. Similarly, an IQ of 85 is one standard deviation below the mean, indicating that only about 14% of people have an IQ lower than this one. Norming a measure makes the values more readily interpretable. Sometimes, but not often, that means they are more readily linked to real-world implications (Blanton & Jaccard, 2006). More likely, it gives a quicker sense of where an observation lies in a distribution of scores without telling us anything about its meaningfulness relative to external (real-world) implications of the score.

Communimetrics seeks to evolve many of the "rules" of psychometric measurement in the design phase. However, as discussed in the chapters that follow, when multiple items are combined to create scale scores, a number of psychometric considerations return as requirements for effective measurement in human service enterprises. It is primarily in the design phase that communimetrics represents a different theory of measurement.

Chapter 3
Designing a Communimetric Measure

As discussed, it is in the design phase that the distinctions between communimetrics and other theories of measurement are the clearest. Psychometric theories of measurement base many major instrument design considerations on the statistical performance of items and sets of items. While statistical relationships can be important, these are not the primary dictates for design considerations of a communimetric tool. This is one reason why some measurement theorists have suggested that clinimetric approaches that focus on the meaning of the item, and psychometric approaches that focus on the statistical performance of the item are complementary (Fava & Belaise, 2005). In this way of thinking, clinimetrics informs the design of items but psychometrics then are performed to determine whether the items are effective.

While clinimetrics offers significant improvements in the meaningfulness of measurement processes to people working within the health care enterprise, it does not take the item design phase far enough in order to maximize the information value within the context of human service enterprises. If you accept the premise that the primary and overriding purpose of measurement in human service enterprise settings is communication, principles of optimizing the communication value of the approach should guide the design process. In other words, the primary goal of a communimetric measurement tool is to effectively communicate the status of one person (or perhaps a family) to other people so that the human service enterprise can be helpful and perhaps even transformative to that person.

The process of designing measurement from classical test theory, item response theory, and clinimetrics have been detailed in a number of excellent resources and are not reviewed here. All measurement development can be thought of as a phased process. There are nine primary phases in the design of a communimetric measurement tool:

1. Define the objectives of measurement.
2. Determine the audiences—those participating in the communication process.
3. Select the items based on what information must be communicated.
4. Create action levels for the items.
5. Develop anchored definitions of each action level for each item.
6. Share draft items with audience representatives and revise according to feedback.

J.S. Lyons, *Communimetrics: A Communication Theory of Measurement in Human Service Settings*,
DOI 10.1007/978-0-387-92822-7_3, © Springer Science+Business Media, LLC 2009

7. Test the tool in a field application.
8. Implement.
9. Repeat the processes in 1 to 6 during the course of the use of the tool.

Phase 1. Defining the Objectives

The process of developing a communimetric tool starts with the specification of the objectives of the tool. While traditional measurement approaches focus on the construct validity of the use, communimetric tools focus on the utility validity (see Chap. 4). Therefore, there is a premium on developing tools that can be simultaneously used for multiple purposes. In most circumstances, it is wise to seek multiple, simultaneous objectives for any tool. By increasing the overall importance of the use of the tool, this multitasking approach helps maximize the utility validity and increases the overall value of the tool.

Most people agree that information supports better decision making; so determining what information is needed and the possible purposes for this information is the challenge of Phase 1 in the measurement development process. The first step of this phase is to decide what information is needed. At this stage the definition of information can be left relatively vague as later phases allow a more detailed fleshing out of the measurement construct. However, at the start it is critical to have a basic conceptualization of the information sought by the measurement process. For example, in designing a tool for employment services one would conceptualize the information needed as factors directly related to employability (e.g., education, job history, job skills) and it likely should be expanded to include factors that might complicate employability (e.g., language and culture, health and behavioral health, functional limitations).

Once the basic domains of information are defined, possible uses should be considered. Table 3.1 contains an example of a basic grid that defines some standard uses of information in human service enterprises. Most settings have at least three levels—the person seeking assistance, the entity providing the help, and the larger

Table 3.1 Examples of Uses of Information at Three Levels of a Market

	Customer	Program or Company	System, Market, or Jurisdiction
Decision support	Service planning	Eligibility	Resource management
	Effective practices	Step-down	Right-sizing
	Evidence-based practices		
Outcome monitoring	Service transitions and celebrations	Program	Provider profiles
		Evaluation	Performance and contracting
Quality improvement	Case management	CQI/QA	Transformation
	Integrated care	Accreditation	Business model design
	Supervision	Program redesign	

system or marketplace in which that transaction occurs. Different types of systems/markets have different names for these components, but all markets have at least these three levels at which information is used. In health care it would be patient, health care professional, hospital, and health care system. In children's services it would be child/family, program, and system of care. In small business incubation it would be entrepreneur, incubator, and market. In corrections it would be prisoner, prison, and jurisdiction. Many markets have much more differentiated levels, but all systems have at least three (i.e., buyer, seller, marketplace).

In addition to the three basic levels of the system, note that Table 3.1 also contains three basic uses of information—decision support, outcomes monitoring and quality improvement. Decision support refers to using information to decide what happens next. This is the most basic and essential use of information in human service enterprises, at least from the perspective of the individual consumer. It is the fundamental application of a communimetric tool. However, beyond the decision support uses for the individual, programs can use information to decide on eligibility. Most programs are designed to benefit specific target populations. A decision support tool that assists in defining who is most likely to benefit from the service enterprise is a program level decision support. Finally, when governmental entities are responsible for systems of programs (or markets), they often need to understand how to "right size" the systems. How do you know whether you have sufficient employment services in the optimal locations? How many hospitals does a health care system need? How many beds in each hospital? Thus, resource management is decision support at the system level.

The second application of information is outcome monitoring. This is the "how are we doing" question. Of course in many businesses, how are we doing often refers to the success of the business financially. The ultimate outcome is profit. Outcomes monitoring, however, is focused on the question of how the enterprise is performing relative to the customer or recipient. It is within this information application that the challenges of managing transformative offerings are most easily recognized. At the individual consumer level an outcome is evidence that a transformation has occurred. More practically it might include determining when to transition to a different program or type of intervention or when to celebrate the end of involvement in the specific enterprise. At the program level, outcomes are a vital component to the well-developed field of program evaluation, which has a large number of its own methods and strategies. In fact, most measurement strategies have arisen historically within the framework of program evaluation. One way to understand the difference between traditional measurement and communimetrics is that traditional measurement starts in the Program Evaluation cell of this grid, while communimetrics starts in the Service Planning cell. Each then works to use the same information across other cells. The system level use of outcomes information includes the emerging strategy of performance contracting (i.e., pay-for-performance). As discussed, human service enterprises remain one of the few industries in which providers are paid regardless of the quality and impact of their work. This situation is not sustainable. Increasingly, people and entities who invest in human services enterprises are developing expectations for how those enterprises should impact the human condition.

Quality improvement involves a large set of strategies for using information to improve the offering (e.g., product, service, or transformation) or the process by which it is delivered. These activities represent the third application of information in human service enterprises. Most enterprises have a quality improvement component, although it is sometimes less formal in human services than in industry. Structured measurement is a key process in quality management, so communimetric tools have many potential applications here as well. At the individual consumer level, examples of quality improvement uses of information include supervision and mentoring new staff and for health and behavioral health services, case management strategies. At the program level, quality improvement is a broad and well-developed set of methods, including such specific strategies as continual quality improvement, quality assurance, total quality management, etc. And at the system level, evolving the quality of the service system is what most people refer to as system transformation.

The list of applications contained in the grid in Table 3.1 is by no means exhaustive. Additional columns exist in some settings (e.g., agencies with multiple programs, regions, systems of multiple program types that interact, and so forth) other uses of information are also possible (e.g., marketing, fund raising). The more applications to which a measurement tool can be applied, the more likely that the tools will prove to be reliable, valid, useful, and sustainable.

Phase 2. Determine the Audiences: Those Participating in the Communication Process

This second phase of measurement development is crucial for achieving a number of critical goals of the measure. After all, the purpose of communication is to express one observation or thought between or among two or more people. The definition of audiences would be anyone who might be involved in sharing and/or using the information contained within the measure. In many ways, determining the audience could be the first phase of the measurement process in communimetrics. The challenge is that it can be quite difficult to engage an audience without a clear purpose so determining the goals and uses first before you engage potential audiences is more efficient and effective.

Clearly, the two audiences that are always involved in the communication are customers and providers. People receiving the offering and people providing the offering are both critical audiences. However, nearly all communimetric measures are designed for multiple audiences beyond these obvious partners. For example, in a health care setting, audiences likely include patients, physicians, nurses, administrators, funders, and policy analysts. In business incubation, audiences may include entrepreneurs, mentors, venture capitalists, and government officials responsible for business growth. In the child serving system, audiences may include youth, parents, siblings, and peers, teachers, counselors, child welfare case workers, probation officers, and more. Effective communication must be understood by all participating audiences.

Therefore, inclusion in the design phase of representatives from each of these target audiences is highly recommended.

A major consideration of this phase of the measurement development is which, if any, audience has precedence over any of the others. If such a hierarchy exists, generally it is recommended that the priority should be given to the audience who will be responsible for completing the measurement process. Thus, for a communimetric measure in health care, priority to physicians and nurses may be indicated, although there may be circumstances in which family or patient preferences are the highest priority. In business incubation, priority to the entrepreneur and his or her mentor may be useful. However, in general, I would recommend that to the extent possible, equal weight is given to all potential audiences in the process of managing the human service enterprise so that the measure becomes a consensus-building approach with every major system partner in agreement on the inclusion of items and the wording of anchored definitions of the action levels, etc.

Of course, there is a difference between having a voice in the development of a tool and having control over that development. Someone (or a small group of people) has to exercise executive control over the process. You cannot develop a tool with a completely inclusive, democratic process. You generally don't get a good product or you never get that product to market when you have too open a development process. Fully democratic processes can become paralyzing. At the same time, you do want all audiences to feel that they had a voice in the process. Research on procedural justice (i.e., Do participants feel the process is fair?) suggests that having a voice in a process is sufficient regardless of whether specific recommendations were followed (Tyler, Rasinski, & Spodick, 1985). Thus, allowing many to participate but reserving the decision making to a limited number of people is an effective process that balances the values of inclusiveness with the need for action and completion. Elsewhere I have referred to this approach as "the illusion of inclusion" (Lyons, 2004). Things do not get done if you always have to reach consensus. You have to allow a voice, but still manage the development process.

There are two key results you want from the partner audiences in the second development phase. First, you would like to build a consensus about the information inputs for the tool. What do people need to know in the specific enterprise applications? For example, if you are communicating about the need for hospitalization, what are the factors to consider in this decision? Second, what words and terms are generally understood within a common framework? You really want to stay away from words that are too trendy or too tied to a specific theory or perspective that is not widely held or likely to fall out of use in a short period of time. For example, in a health care application in the United States you would probably hesitate to include references to meridians. However, if the health care application were within a traditional Chinese setting, such concepts might be relevant. Similarly in mental health there are a number of competing theories of behavior. You would prefer that your instrument does not pick sides in any theoretical disputes unless the tool is to be used only within one theory's treatment approach. One of the great advantages of including all audiences in the early stages of development is that you will quickly learn which words are too tied to a controversial position or approach or are simply unacceptable to certain audiences.

A great example of this process comes from the development of the CANS (see Chap. 5). The original version of the tool was develop based on partner audience-focused discussions, but not vetted back to those audiences. The first version of the tool, called the Childhood Severity of Psychiatric Illness (CSPI), used several terms that can be experienced as offensive by certain audiences. For example, the word *illness* in the title of the tool emphasized a medical model that made some parents and non-physician mental health professionals uncomfortable. Further several of the items used the term *dysfunction*. This word is offensive to some parents and to professionals who are strength-based in their approach. Calling something functioning is OK. Calling functioning problems *dysfunction* alienates certain potential partners.

There are multiple methods of audience participation. My favored approach is focus groups. Ideally, focus groups that combine different audience representatives are effective. However, some thought should be put into whether one audience might be silenced by another. That is, some audiences may intimidate other audiences. For example, unless you have pretty courageous patient representatives they will often defer to physicians in combined groups. Care should be taken to determine whether this concern is operable across your selected audiences. If that is a concern, separate groups for separate audiences are recommended.

In terms of methods for focus group participation there are many choices. Qualitative researchers have developed a series of sophisticated strategies to obtain and analyze information from focus group discussions (e.g., Kitzinger, 1994; Krueger & Casey, 2000) These methods might involve taping and transcribing the session and analyzing the text with sophisticated computerized tools. In my experience, you do not need these methods in order to obtain the information you need to move forward with the design of the instrumentation. Although it might be a good idea to tape the sessions in case you can't keep good notes. However, if you are seeking external funding or planning to try to publish your work in a peer-reviewed scientific journal, adherence to a higher level of methodological rigor will be important.

Phase 3. Selecting Items

Once you have established the objectives of the measurement process and the audience who will be communicating with each other about the object of measurement, the next step in designing a measure is to select the individual items for inclusion. Communimetric tools are designed to have single items that can stand alone and be useful. Therefore, the selection of items is generally guided by the concept of what needs to be communicated as an output of a measurement or assessment process.

The primary principle of item selection is to determine what information you need to make good decisions in whatever human service settings you seek to facilitate. Thus, the use of the tool in terms of supporting decision making at the individual level should drive its design. All things that are relevant to service and intervention planning should be included. Things that do not vary or are irrelevant to the service planning process should not be included. Start with an understanding of the initial assessment and planning process. What information is routinely collected? How is it related to intervention planning processes? What are the intervention choices? What factors make intervention more difficult?

Part of the decision about items selection is also level of measurement. It is at this point in the design that one should consider at what level the items should be used. One can create items at a global level (e.g., intelligence, depression) or at a more molecular level (e.g., math problem solving, sleep disruption). The level of the measurement should be consistent with the level of the decision making to be made at the individual level. Each item will eventually map into a different potential action. One should generally avoid having to combine items to suggest a specific action, as that logic will require scoring before the measure can be useful at the individual level. The exceptions to this rule are program eligibility strategies that invariably require decision models that combine multiple items into some form of a severity or complexity model.

Often it is useful to start with potential actions and work backward to determine what information is needed to decide whether or not to take a specific available option. For example, if you are providing housing services and you do not have any links to mental health care, it might be irrelevant to include any items in your tool that describe mental health needs unless you are trying to identify gaps in the existing system. However, if you have options of referral (or better yet, integrated care) to a mental health treatment program that works collaboratively with the housing program, then it is quite useful to include an item or items on mental health needs, as that information can inform potential action choices.

It has been my experience that focus group methods are quite helpful in this phase as well. Often one can use the results of Phase 2 focus groups to inform this phase of the developmental process. Key partner interviews are reasonable, but less efficient, alternatives. The process of selecting items then is to identify which inputs are relevant to the potential outputs at all levels.

Other sources for identifying potential items include the review of the scientific literature, personal experience with assessment and service delivery and systematic review of existing records from the service delivery system. This later method is an intriguing one in that the review of information sources such as medical charts, and personnel files can often give a sense of what information is currently deemed relevant to the service delivery operation. The downside of the approach is that it is often difficult to do a file review without already having a draft of the tool (see the following) or at least having a clear idea of what you are looking for in the review process. I generally use file review methods as a form of rapid piloting in the field (see Phase 7).

Phase 4. Create Action Levels for the Items

This is the step in the design of the communimetric tool intended to ensure that the measurement process is not arbitrary (Blanton & Jaccard, 2006). Here you work to tie the levels of individual items to real-world consequences of the information with the regard to actions in the human service enterprise. Creating the action levels will depend in large part of the activity informed by the measurement. The simplest communimetric scale would be the following:

1. Don't do it.
2. Do it.

This two-level scale distinguishes action from inaction. It is the simplest metric that at some level describes all decisions related to human behavior. Of course, humans are often more nuanced in debating whether or not to act.

If you were planning on cleaning your refrigerator and you want a decision support tool, you might consider the following action levels:

0 The food is still good.
1 It is nearing expiration, better eat it soon.
2 It has expired. You should probably pitch it unless you're desperate.
3 It looks and smells awful. Throw it out now before someone sees what you have in your refrigerator or you make yourself sick.

An accountant friend of mine suggested the following tongue-in-cheek accounting action level scale:

0 No tax audit
1 Minor tax audit
2 Major tax audit
3 Prison time

Perhaps it becomes rapidly clear that any set of actions can be used to create a communimetric scale. The most commonly used scale is the following:

0 No evidence, no need for action
1 Watchful waiting/prevention (Keep an eye on it.)
2 Action
3 Immediate or Intensive Action

This is the scale used in the CANS, the INTERMED, and the ELSA as described in later chapters. This scale works well for needs or problems or challenges that will be addressed through intervention. The CANS also has items that assess strengths. The following action levels are used:

0 Centerpiece strength—focus of a strength-based plan
1 Useful strength—can be included in a strength based plan
2 Identified strength—must be built before use
3 No strength identified

An action level model that can be used for items in a strategic planning process could be structured as follows:

0 Not included
1 Parking lot (consider later)
2 Include
3 Make a priority

With this scale a set of action items would be identified during a brainstorming session, and then the group could assign action levels based on the preceding rating scale. The items could be organized by priority.

Here's an example of a possible action scale for a mastery assessment:

0 No skill evident, needs to develop skill
1 Remedial skill level, needs some help
2 Competent, able to perform skill adequately
3 Proficient/skilled, expert at performing skill

A set of learning or mastery skills could be identified, and then an individual could be assessed on each skill. A profile of ratings would be a map of what skills must be developed and where skill strengths exist.

Phase 5. Develop Anchored Definitions of Action Levels for Each Item

Once the items and action levels are determined, it is necessary to describe the construct assessed at each of the selected item levels. This phase of the tool development requires the most working knowledge of the field to which the measure is to be applied. Creating short definitions for each action level grounds the measure by translating characteristics of the construct covered by the item into action levels within the proposed context of use of the tool. In other words, the goal of the anchored definitions is to translate levels of an item into words that describe the levels of the construct that would indicate different levels of action.

The following is an example item from the Child and Adolescent Needs and Strengths for children and youth with mental health challenges (CANS-MH). This item is designed to communicate the level of suicidality of the person described. The CANS-MH uses 0 no evidence, 1 watchful waiting/prevention, 2 action, and 3 immediate or intensive action.

Danger to Self

This rating describes both suicidal and significant self-injurious behavior. A rating of 2 or 3 would indicate the need for a safety plan.

0 Child has no evidence or history of suicidal behaviors
1 History of suicidal behaviors, but no suicidal behavior during the past 30 days
2 Recent (last 30 days) but not acute (today) suicidal ideation or gesture
3 Current suicidal ideation and intent in the past 24 hours

Notice that the 0 level includes both no current evidence and no history. This is because a history of significant suicidal behavior is a risk factor for future behavior and thus would increase the person to a watchful waiting/prevention action level. A history of suicidal behavior would be rated a 1. Recent ideation or gesture would be actionable in that a safety plan would be developed and it would be directly addressed in treatment. Acute suicidal ideation and intent warrants immediate action, and psychiatric hospitalization might be considered. Consequently, the design of the anchored definitions is designed to be consistent with what we know about best practices of addressing suicidal risk.

Understanding the meaning of history in the watchful/waiting prevention rating level is important. History should be understood as history that is relevant to the present. So, having transient suicidal thoughts may not last as historically important for very long, while trying to hang oneself might be included as a history of suicidal behavior for a lifetime.

Here is a different item structure from the same tool.

Antisocial Behavior (Compliance with Society's Rules)

These symptoms include antisocial behaviors like shoplifting, lying, vandalism, cruelty to animals, and assault. This dimension would include the symptoms of Conduct Disorder as specified in DSM-IV.

0 This rating indicates a child with no evidence of behavior disorder.
1. This rating indicates a child with a mild level of conduct problems. Some antisocial behavior in school and/or home. Problems recognizable but not notably deviant for age, sex, and community. This might include occasional truancy, lying, or petty theft from family.
2. This rating indicates a child with a moderate level of conduct disorder. This could include episodes of planned aggression or other antisocial behavior. A child rated at this level should meet the criteria for a diagnosis of Conduct Disorder.
3. This rating indicates a child with a severe Conduct Disorder. This could include frequent episodes of unprovoked, planned aggression or other antisocial behavior.

In this item, the anchored definitions are actually tied to an alternative measurement scheme that is commonly used in mental health—the Diagnostic and Statistical Manual (DSM-IVTR, APA, 2004). While the item is not diagnostic, it is consistent with diagnoses. In DSM, a diagnosis is defined as symptoms that led to dysfunction or distress. This conceptualization translates into actionable needs in a communimetric framework (i.e., ratings of 2 or 3). A rating of 1 might be consistent with a diagnosis of rule out/in or in remission or a subthreshold set of symptoms that do not quite rise to the level of diagnostic criteria.

In the design of the anchored definitions, a balance must be sought. Enough information should be provided so that people completing the tool will have a reasonably clear sense of how to translate information about the status of the item with an individual into action levels. At the same time it is important not to provide too much information. I generally recommend one to three sentences for each action level in the anchors.

The danger of too much information is that it might limit the raters. For example, it is likely impossible to completely describe all possible presentations of suicidal behavior and risk with a four-level anchored rating scale no matter how long those descriptions were allowed to run. Too much information encourages raters to be concrete and look for a completely accurate match in the anchors of the person they are working to describe. Often, people defy such easy categorization; therefore, flexibility must be built into the rating system. For example, you may note that no mention of preoccupation with death is mentioned in the anchored definitions for suicide. Now, in many cases, a child or youth who appears to be preoccupied with death would warrant close monitoring, which would imply a 1 rating. However, there may be extreme circumstances that the preoccupation rises to the level that requires therapeutic intervention or safety planning, which would be a 2 rating. By using the action levels as the ultimate trumps communimetric tool allows the person completing the measure the flexibility to best communicate service needs within a context of varied and potentially complex presentations.

For the same reason, I recommend avoiding the use of examples in the anchored definitions to the extent possible. Examples bring the levels to life in important ways by providing raters with stories to help them understand the words. This process is quite valuable in training. However, when specific examples are included in the anchors, some raters become quite concrete and the only people they will rate at a specific level will be those who fit the specific example provided. One useful strategy is to put examples in a glossary that is a supplementary document to the manual. That way detailed examples can be given for those who are working to understand the levels of the items, but they are not in the rating definitions that are used day-to-day. Including examples in training is critical to a successful training. The glossary works more as a training aid while the manual is more of a work aid.

Phase 6. Share Draft Items for Feedback from Audience Representatives

It is an important phase in the design to take the draft version of the now existing tool to share with representatives of the audiences that participated back in Phase 2. Return to the target audiences is important for two reasons. First, it is helpful to ensure that you heard them correctly and got their input accurately as you developed the tool in the Phases following Phase 2. It is possible to get derailed during the subsequent Phases and drift away from the original communication purpose. Also, the creation of the anchored ratings may not have been reviewed by target audiences until this point. Feedback from these audiences generally focuses on the naming of items or the definition of action levels. Sometimes once a full draft is developed, item inclusion or exclusion also should be reconsidered. Using the same or overlapping audience representatives is generally recommended for two reasons. First, they already have had the project explained so the second meeting is more efficient. Second, often members think about their experience in the first meeting and have new ideas developed at the follow-up meeting. This experience over time adds depth to the item development process that would be less available with one-shot exposures to target audience members.

The second value of returning to the audiences for feedback is the sociopolitical advantages that come from an inclusive process with key partners who will be using the tool involved. Phases 2 and 6 together allow a measure developer to argue that standards of inclusion were met and that people had an opportunity for input into the process (regardless of whether they chose to exercise that opportunity).

The specific method to obtain feedback can vary. In some settings it is useful to reconvene focus groups and review the tool together in an open forum. The advantage of this approach is that people in group often feed off of each other in terms of stimulating ideas and reactions. Feedback from these groups can be quite informative. The disadvantages include they are more time consuming and can be difficult to manage productively. If you decide to convene groups, the same issues arise here as in Phase 2.

Sometimes it is more convenient to simply distribute the draft tool electronically and ask for people to comment within a designated time period. If you have an on-board target audience, virtual meetings are sufficient. If you have to worry about the degree to which the audience supports the measurement development process, face-to-face meetings are recommended.

Phase 7. Test the Tool in a Field Application

Pilot testing is an essential component to the implementation of any process. It is only by actually attempting to use the tool that many possible opportunities and barriers are identified. The optimal way to pilot a measure is to use it in precisely the manner that you hope to use it at full implementation. This may be an impossible goal but one worthy to approximate. In some cases, a pilot can be used to test different implementation strategies. In general, a pilot should be designed to address at least the following questions:

- Can representatives of the target population of raters be trained to use the tool reliably?
- Is the information requested by the tool available at the time the tool is to be completed?
- Can the tool be completed in a timely fashion without disrupting work flow?
- Can the tool be integrated into the work itself so that it is useful?
- How do people who participate in its completion find it?
- How do consumers and recipients find it?

If the piloting concern is more about the structure of the tool than its use, then a different form of piloting can be useful. Since communimetric tools are designed as information integration strategies, it is sometimes possible to include a record review as a component of the pilot process (Lyons, Mintzer, Kisiel, & Shallcross, 1998). Use of file review methods is a time- and cost-effective method for piloting and can provide very useful information about the fit of the information included in the measure with information that is routinely collected in the service delivery setting that is being reviewed. File reviews can also be used to begin to validate the tool in terms of its relationship with intervention planning and program eligibility decisions.

A key assumption in the file review process is that no mention represents no evidence. This assumption is similar to a key quality assurance assumption for chart audits in health care, "If it isn't documented; it doesn't exist." Assuming that all relevant needs or strengths are documented if identified allows the file review process to indicate what needs and strengths have been used in the process of care, even with relatively scant records. We have demonstrated that information collected in file review using communimetric tools is validly associated with prospectively collected measures (Lyons, 2004; Lyons, Colletta, Devens, & Finkel, 1995).

Phase 8. Implement

Implementation of any measurement process in human service delivery enterprises can be a very complex undertaking. Human services providers may not be used to completing measures, or they may have had bad experiences or gotten into bad habits with prior measures, or they might just begrudge that someone is asking them to do something that they may feel is just more work with no relevance to them or their work.

After piloting, there are usually three basic approaches to implementation:

- Immediate widespread
- Planned incremental
- Individual/gradual

Immediate widespread implementation involves picking a date at which time everyone in the target service system is expected to begin using the tool. Planned incremental implementation is a step-by-step process in which segments of the target service system implement sequentially. Individual and gradual implementation is simply making the tool available and seeing who chooses to use it.

Immediate Widespread

This form of implementation is easiest from an administrative perspective—e.g., "everybody starts today"—and the greatest challenge is to actually succeed in widespread effective use of the tool. I sometimes refer to this as the Iraqi strategy. The U.S invasion of Iraq to dethrone Saddam Hussein was rapid, but the process of cleaning up the chaos that the invasion caused was difficult, complex, and messy. The main problem with immediate widespread implementation is that the process of supporting training and good utilization is very difficult to do evenly and the process of cleaning up the implementation can lead to what could be called implementation fatigue. Sometimes, failures in implementation get blamed on the tool itself, when the problem is actually a challenge with training or operations.

The major advantage of the immediate and widespread implementation process is that if you have a narrow political window for an implementation to occur it is sometimes useful to force it as far as possible in order to make it irreversible for others who follow. This is a strategy favored by political appointees. In North America and Europe there are generally two sectors in the bureaucracy: the political bureaucracy and the permanent bureaucracy. The political bureaucrats are appointed by the current government and have relatively short tenures in any given position. The permanent bureaucracy is populated by career bureaucrats who outlive most political appointees in their positions. The goal of the political bureaucracy is to establish a vision and drive it as far into the permanent bureaucracy as possible during their relatively short tenure. For this reason, they favor an immediate, widespread implementation strategy. Of course, that leads members of the permanent bureaucracy to sometimes see things as the flavor of the month, or something that will go away if you just ignore it.

Planned Incremental

The counterpoint to the Iraqi strategy is the South African strategy. The world community placed sanctions on South Africa because of their egregious civil rights abuses during apartheid. Over time with this pressure, the South African government eventually relented and apartheid was ended. This is an example of a planned incremental strategy. Planned incrementalism is a paced approach to implementation that tries to roll out a tool in a sequential fashion that establishes its utility and effectiveness first in smaller settings before encouraging its use more broadly.

As an example, the Illinois Department of Children and Family Services (IDCFS) is using the CANS throughout its system. The first implementation was in 2002 as a planning and outcome tool in their foster care stabilization program. Then, in 2004, it was begun to be used in the residential treatment system to monitor outcomes for children and youth in the most intensive and expensive placements. Next, in 2005, the CANS was implemented in the Integrated Assessment, which occurs for all children and youth at entry into IDCFS custody. The next implementation, also in 2005, occurred with the Child and Youth Investment Teams (CAYIT), which are used to make decisions about placement if a child or youth is thought to need something beyond regular foster care. In 2009, it began to be used at the Administrative Case Reviews that occur for all children and youth every 6 months during their stay with IDCFS.

The advantage of planned incrementalism is that it provides a natural process for adjusting and evolving the tool to make sure it supports the work. Feedback from early experiences can be used to adjust either the tool itself or the process by which it is used. Planned incrementalism also can reduce resistance by building positive experiences that can be used as examples for later implementations (e.g., "See, they did it and found it helpful."). The disadvantage is if you have a segment of the system that is highly resistant, an incremental approach may lead to a longer overall struggle against this type of entrenched resistance. Despite this challenge, my experience suggests that planned incremental approaches have greater long-term sustainability (Lyons, 2004).

Individual/Gradual

This implementation strategy is the only available approach if the tool is not a required activity within a particular service delivery system. If use of the tool is entirely voluntary, then the implementation strategy looks more like a marketing/sales strategy than the other two approaches. To date, most communimetric tools have been implemented initially in this individual/gradual fashion by referral (i.e., word of mouth). Someone is exposed to the tool, uses it, likes it, and then talks to someone else about it. To my knowledge, no communimetric tool has ever been actively advertised or marketed, and yet the use of these tools is quite widespread, suggesting that word of mouth from satisfied users is a powerful support for implementation.

Frequently individual/gradual implementations set the groundwork for system-wide implementations. The State of Indiana went statewide with both the CANS and the adult version, the Adult Needs and Strengths Assessment (ANSA) after individual counties and several large providers had begun using the tools. Since a notable part of the system partners were already using the tools and happy with them, this made the implementation of the statewide approach somewhat easier, or at least more palpable.

Sometimes it is possible to use an immediate/widespread implementation strategy with planned incrementalism. In this strategy, the completion of the tool is immediate and widespread; everyone starts completing it at the same time. Applications of the tool (e.g., decision support for specific programs) are then implemented incrementally. This approach is quite useful when there is a strong history of people using a prior tool for advocacy rather than accuracy. In other words, if people have been completing a prior tool in a certain way to guarantee a certain outcome (e.g., funding for a specific service), it is valuable to use a two-stage process to break this destructive habit. First, you get people used to using the new tool and emphasize the accuracy (i.e., reliability) with which they used it. Then, after you've worked to establish a culture of accuracy, you implement those applications that have been historically drive by covert agendas, such as funding or other considerations.

Working the Organization

The implementation of the communimetric tools should not be exclusively about reaching full use penetration (i.e., everybody using it). While getting target individuals and groups to actually complete the measure is one aspect of effective implementation, sustained use will likely require not just embracing the form but at least recognizing the utility of the measure as a tool and, perhaps, ultimately accepting its use as a framework. Therefore, there is a component of all implementation processes that could be considered "working the organization." Somebody (or multiple people) must champion this change and enthusiastically support it and explain to the people who must participate in the measurement process the value of that participation.

Rosen and Weil (1996) describe three types of employees when it comes to reactions to innovation. The first types are referred to as Eager Adopters (others use the term Early Adopters). These are the individuals who are first on board any new thing. They buy the latest technology. They pride themselves on being on the cutting edge. Estimates range that between 10% and 15% of the work force are eager adopters. They provide the energy and enthusiasm for any change process.

In most work places, the largest group is what Rosen and Weil term Hesitant-Prove-Its. They function with the philosophy that as soon as you show me this is of some benefit (preferably to me, but at least to my work), then I'm on board. These folks tend to be skeptical. A hands-on demonstration of the utility of the approach is often required before they are convinced to get on the bus. Rosen and Weil suggest about 70% to 80% of the work force falls into this type. Efforts generally must focus on these individuals, because the success of the implementation generally depends on whether these workers see and experience the utility of the tool.

The final type of worker is what the authors refer to as Resistors. These individuals refuse to change. They will fight the implementation openly or sabotage it if open resistance is not feasible. Generally, only job sanctions work with these workers. The percent of resistors varies by setting from 10% to 15%.

A strategy we have used in a number of settings to facilitate a system's willingness and ability to embrace a philosophical shift has been the development of agency- or program-based champions. These individuals are trained to instruct others in the use of the measure, but they are also asked to provide training, supervision, and support to use the measure in all of its relevant applications in their place of employment. In a number of jurisdictions we have referred to these champions as Super Users.

Super User Programs

We have used what have been called Super Users to assist in the process of implementing several communimetric tools, specifically the CANS and ANSA (see Chap. 5) in the field. As discussed, the theory of communimetric measurement is to not stop with the concept of the measure itself, but rather to create an environment in which the measurement can be at least a tool to assist people in the field in successfully completing their work or, ideally, a framework; that is, the communimetric measure becoming the work.

There are many challenges to shifting field workers away from thinking of a measure as a form to be completed in considering it a tool or framework. There is a substantial amount of research that suggests that having role model or champions for a particular skill or approach facilitates changes in work (Olson, Eoyard, Beckard, & Vaill, 2001) There is also a body of research that demonstrates that people are more likely to listen to people who are more similar to them in terms of advice about change processes (Shaw, 2002). In the Super User model, staff members are identified at participating programs and/or agencies. These staff members are developed as trainers in the reliable completion of the measure, but they are also taught the multiple applications of the measure so that programs/agencies are better able to fully use the measure in all of its applications (see Chap. 5). If done correctly, the Super Users become ambassadors to the implementation process.

In general, Super User programs start with the initial widespread implementation of the tool. Initially, Super Users are trained to either provide training in the reliable use of the measure or support training and certification processes if those are offered online or provided through other centralized strategies. The reliability requirements to become a Super Users are generally higher than those required to become certified in the use of the tool. Super Users are given additional training in training strategies and curriculum. However, the Super User cohort should not stop simply at becoming trainers. Through the use of e-mail and regular (e.g., quarterly) meetings, additional skill sets are developed so that the Super Users can take back to program/agency staff various applications of the measure. For example, with the CANS we have provided Super User groups with additional training in strength-based planning, quality improvement approaches, and outcomes monitoring/ program evaluation approaches.

Phase 9. Repeat the Processes in Phases 1 to 6 During the Course of Service Delivery

Unlike a research tool that can be viewed as sacrosanct once it has been developed (i.e., change the items and you change the reliability and validity of the measure), a communimetric tool is intended to be fluid—much like communication itself. The reason anyone might use a communimetric tool within a service delivery system would be to support improvements in that system. Therefore, the tool must be held to precisely the same standard. If experiences require the addition or deletion of items or a change in the wording of an item anchor, then that should be accomplished. Of course, you want to accomplish changes in an organized, systematic manner. More importantly, though, you want to plan for changes in the tool.

Since communimetric tools are organized at the item level, this creates a situation in which the edit of a measure has less impact on a legacy database than similar changes made to a psychometrically designed measure. Items that remain consistent across versions could still be used to understand changes over time. Consequently, version 2.0 can easily be compared with version 1.0 on the common items.

Most large-scale implementations have scheduled times for revisions. Generally, there is a promise of no change in the tool for the first year or two of its use. During this period, people gain experience and develop an understanding of the approach and work to fully embed it in the human service enterprise. Sometimes small changes occur more rapidly. Particularly if any aspect of an initial version is simply wrong (e.g., referring to Tourette's disease as a developmental disorder) that mistake can just be edited out of the manual. But adding or deleting or dramatically changing items requires a more thoughtful process. Often, issues that arise are not really with the design of the tool but with training in its use. Allowing some time prior to revision allows most of these issues to be resolved through more effective training.

Building Decision Models

A common application of communimetric measures is decision support. Individual level planning to address specific needs is generally done at the item level and usually combinations of items are unnecessary for this type of decision support. However, when the effort is to support decisions regarding program or placement referrals then the decision models are often more complicated and require the involvement of multiple items.

Most traditional measurement approaches create aggregate scores and thus use cutoffs to provide decision support. This strategy is problematic in that it views the characteristics that inform decisions about program or placement as falling on a continuum. Often, that is not how actual decisions are made. Rather, decision making for program or placement referrals often look at profiles of needs across various dimensions. The logic can be Boolean rather than linear. In other words, decisions might have branching logic rather than linear combinations of predictors. Many decisions are actually informed by patterns of needs.

For that reason, decision support models (or algorithms, as some call them) are generated as patterns of actionable items. For example, Table 3.2 provides a decision model used for treatment foster care referrals in Philadelphia. Notice that the model can be described clinically. First, the child either has to have an actionable developmental need or an actionable behavioral health need. They need to have something to treat to justify treatment foster care. However, just those needs could be adequately addressed with an outpatient referral. To justify the use of a therapeutic living environment, additional complications are necessary—functioning disabilities, severe school or social behavior problems, or actionable risk behaviors.

Decision Support Strategies

Two strategies exist for decision support applications—eligibility approaches and quality improvement approaches. In the first approach, the tool is used prospectively to either make or inform a decision. In the latter approach, the tool is used to report back on decision-making performance. Each has advantages and disadvantages,

Table 3.2 Philadelphia Department of Human Services Thresholds for Eligibility for Treatment Foster Care (TFC) Based on the Child and Adolescent Needs and Strengths (CANS)

Criterion	Area	Rating	CANS item
1—Diagnosis	Presence of two or more symptom areas associated with a serious emotional/ behavioral disorder	2 or 3	17. Psychosis 18. Attention deficit/impulse control 19. Depression/anxiety 20. Anger control 21. Oppositional behavior 22. Antisocial behavior 23. Adjustment to trauma 24. Attachment 33. Severity of substance abuse
2—Functioning	Notable impairment in functioning in at least one area	3	1. Motor 2. Sensory 3. Intellectual 4. Communication 5. Developmental 6. Self-care/daily living skills 7. Physical/medical
3—School	Notable impairment in school functioning	3	9. School achievement 10. School behavior 11. School attendance
4—Risk A	Notable risk behaviors in at least one these areas	2 or 3	29. Danger to self 30. Fire setting 31. Runaway 38. Seriousness of criminal behavior 41. Sexually abusive behavior
5—Risk B	Notable risk behaviors in at least one of these areas	"3"	30. Social behavior 40. Violence

In order for a child/youth to be deemed eligible for TFC, she or he must score the following:
The child or youth must have at least TWO 2s or 3s for Criterion 1—Diagnosis AND
a 2 or 3 for Criterion 2—Functioning OR
a 3 for Criterion 3—School OR
a 2 or 3 for Criterion 4—Risk A OR a 3 for Criterion 5—Risk B.

and your choice should be based on the specific circumstances that you hope to influence through the introduction of decision support.

Eligibility Models

In this form of decision support, the tool is utilized before the decision is made. The results of the tool are used to inform the decision. In other words, the tool can be used to determine eligibility to different treatments or levels of care. The basic logic of the approach as outlined in Lyons & Weiner (2009) is to use the following step-wise process:

1. Select and develop a measure that captures the essential information that should be ideally used to make the target decision.
2. Test the measure on a sample of cases to ensure that it identifies the target population as defined by the following characteristics:
   a. Has the clinical characteristics for which the program is intended
   b. Has evidence that these individual actually benefit from receipt of the program or intervention
   c. Does not overly disrupt existing service enterprise by creating radically different decisions; i.e., not radically different than the current wisdom of the field
3. Develop the decision support model on the sample described in the preceding.
4. Pilot the model with new cases to ensure that it works in the field in a way that is consistent with it design intentions.
5. Design an easy, efficient, and fair appeal process for disagreement among partners in the process about the recommended decision.
6. Implement, Monitor, and Adjust.

Eligibility models of decision support can have a transformational effect on an existing service system by creating greater consistency, reducing errors, and subsequently improving outcomes. The challenge of an eligibility model is that in some circumstances it may be perceived as encouraging cookie cutter thinking. Clinical brilliance is the ability to recognize something unique about a person and his or her situation that leads you to do something different than what would be typical. Eligibility systems can discourage clinical brilliance. Thus, establishing appeal processes is an important aspect of managing an eligibility model. In most of our implementations, appeals run about 2% to 5%, depending on the maturity of the system (i.e., more mature systems have fewer appeals).

An example of an eligibility model in the general hospital would be any case that involves an automatic referral. For example, an automatic referral to Consultation/Liaison (C/L) Psychiatry for a drug overdose is a simple example of an eligibility model. Once the assessment is made that the patient has experienced a drug overdose, then a referral is made. The C/L psychiatrist or nurse practitioner takes it from there. The INTERMED approach can be used for this type of eligibility referral (see Chap. 6). The presence of any specific actionable need can generate an automatic referral.

Patterns of actionable needs could be used for the intensity of approach. These patterns are the algorithms described in the preceding, such as demonstrated in Table 3.2. Creating algorithms for eligibility models is accomplished with the same method with an effort to identify those individuals most likely to benefit from the target program or interventions.

Quality Improvement Models

In this second approach to decision support, the tool is completed at the time of the decision, but no analysis or interpretation is done at that time and no recommendation is made to the deciding clinicians. Rather, feedback is given to these clinicians after a period of time has passed. Using an emergency department process as an example, this feedback could be both individual (e.g., You admitted John to the hospital when most people would not. Why?) or in aggregate (e.g., percent of low risk admissions and percent of high-risk deflections).

We have used the Severity of Psychiatric Illness (SPI) in a variety of settings for this type of quality improvement models. Items from the SPI can be used to generate a predictive model of psychiatric admission (Lyons, Kisiel, Dulcan, Cohen, & Chesler 1997; Mulder et al., 2000) and readmission (Lyons et al., 1997). These models identify those patients most likely to benefit by hospitalization. They also can be used to understand patterns of utilization (Yohanna et al., 2000). Once established, these models can be used to understand other factors that interfere with good practice (Mulder et al., 2005).

A variety of strategies can be used to establish models—either clinical or statistical. The clinical strategies involve using the communimetric tool to define the target populations. For example, for a psychiatric hospitalization sample, you might say that a patient with a 3 (immediate/intensive action) on the following items:

- Psychosis
- Danger to self
- Danger to others
- Self-care

and a combination of 2 (i.e., actionable) on any three would describe a target population for psychiatric hospital admission. Further, you could add a 2 on Psychosis with a 3 on Medication Compliance. As you can see, the communimetric measurement approach is a very natural fit to a clinical decision support model, and it naturally divides things out from an action perspective.

Statistical approaches generally involve either the use of logistic regression (for two category decisions—admit/not admit) or discriminant function analysis (for three or more category decisions). In these models, a development sample is collected where the decision support tool is collected in the natural environment along with the decision made (unsupported by the assessment). This development sample is used to calculate the statistical relationship between the items of the assessment and the actual decision (cf., Lyons, 2004; Lyons et al., 1997). A prediction model is generated from these data. Next, it is important to test the model on a validation sample of about the same size. This is critical in that most statistical approaches maximize the relationship in the development stage and some shrinkage in the prediction accuracy should be expected when the model is applied to a new sample. Too much shrinkage invalidates the original model.

Summary

This chapter highlights the design process recommended for the creation of a communimetric measure. The precise process used, like the tool itself, depends in great part on the context of the human service enterprise for which it is to be used.

This chapter clarifies that the core of communimetrics is to understand what aspects of the person must be communicated in order to support good decisions that lead to effective interventions. This perspective is not really different than what developers of psychometric tools would say. What is different is that once identified, this information is placed into an action-oriented structure that supports individual-level decision making while allowing applications at other levels and in other sectors of the market or system. The next chapter discusses how you might know you have been successful in enhancing communication through the use of measurement in the target enterprise.

Chapter 4
Defining a "Good" Communimetric Measurement Tool: Reliability and Validity Considerations

The quality of any measurement process is defined by at least two essential characteristics—the consistency and accuracy with which the measurement process can be applied and the degree to which the measure is capturing the construct or constructs it is purported to measure. These two related measurement characteristics are commonly referred to as reliability and validity. Given the design approach of a communimetric measurement tool, considerations regarding reliability and validity are distinct but overlapping depending on the use to which the tool is applied. For analyses of aggregated data in which the tool is scored by dimensions, the concepts of reliability and validity are very consistent with traditional psychometric consideration. However, for other applications, the unique characteristics of a communimetric measure require an elaboration of additional considerations about both reliability and validity.

Reliability

Reliability is the accuracy of a measure: To what degree can you repeat a measurement operation and expect to get identical results? Reliability is a critical characteristic of all measures. It is necessary but not sufficient to define a good measure. There are three types of reliability to consider when evaluating a measure in traditional psychometric approaches: internal consistency, test-retest, and inter-rater reliability.

Internal consistency reliability refers to the degree to which multiple items on a tool correlate with each other. Cronbach's alpha (Cronbach, 1951) is the accepted standard measure of internal consistency, although historically, split-half reliability was also used (i.e., the correlation of one half of the items to the other half). Cronbach's alpha is conceptually, although not technically, the average of all possible split halves. Internal consistency reliability is quite useful for measures designed to assess internal transient states that are not observable. If the person reporting is the only person with access to the necessary information (e.g., How do I feel?), and that information can easily change over time, then internal consistency is the only reasonable method to gauge reliability. The idea is that by triangulating measurement

J.S. Lyons, *Communimetrics: A Communication Theory of Measurement in Human Service Settings*,
DOI 10.1007/978-0-387-92822-7_4, © Springer Science+Business Media, LLC 2009

of an unobservable, transient construct across multiple items, one can simultaneously achieve and estimate reliability. This idea, of course, requires that all your items actually do measure the same construct, so there is a bit of circularity to the logic of internal consistency reliability. To be reliable you have to have a set of items from the same construct correlate with each other, but you only know that they are from the same construct because they do, in fact, correlate with each other.

Test–retest reliability is calculated by correlating a score on a test at time 1 with the score on the test at time 2. This reliability estimate is a good way of assessing the stability of a measure. It is ideal for measures of constructs that are not expected to change much over time. Of course, you have to worry about practice effects and other sorts of threats to the accurate estimation of this type of reliability when you are repeating the same measurement operations in fairly close sequence. Generally, a 1- or 2-week difference between time one and time two is recommended, but this depends somewhat on the characteristics of the measure and nature of the construct(s). It is interesting that in the science of test-retest reliability there is some notion that it is a good thing if the people assessed do not remember the time 1 assessment (Anastasi, 1968; Nunally, 1976)—the less salient the better for estimating test-retest reliability. This notion is ironic in the context of human service enterprises in which you are probably attempting to measure things that really matter to people (i.e., That's why they are seeking help.). A traditionalist might argue that such an importance would lead to an overestimation of reliability using test-retest reliability. From a communimetrics perspective, such an argument would be a symptomatic of a misunderstanding of the role of measurement in these settings. Of course, someone seeking help from a human service enterprise would just wonder, "Why are you asking me again? You already asked me this question."

Inter-rater reliability is calculated by correlating scores between two raters (or among multiple raters). This reliability estimate is a good way of monitoring whether different people are completing the measure in the same way. This strategy is only possible when the information used to complete the measure involves observable phenomena. The complexities of inter-rater reliability involve methodological controls over what is observable.

In communimetrics, inter-rater reliability is far and away the most important means of estimating the accuracy of the measure. The very nature of communication involves multiple parties, and ensuring that they are using the language of the measure in comparable ways is critical to the integrity of the approach. Internal consistency reliability has a limited and specific role in the measurement model. Depending on the phenomenon being measured, test-retest reliability is close to irrelevant. Let's review each type of reliability in greater detail as it applies to communimetrics.

Internal Consistency

This form of reliability is primarily used for multiple item scales to ensure that each item is measuring the same underlying construct. It is particularly useful when measuring transient internal states (e.g., mood) because only one person has access to the information sought for the measurement operation (i.e., the person experiencing the mood) and it is likely to change over time (i.e., moods shift rapidly with events, blood sugar levels, time of day, etc). Thus, having multiple separate measurement operations (i.e., multiple items on a single measure) are thought to allow us to approximate reliability by assessing the degree to which these multiple operations give the same measurement results. The most common statistic applied for this purpose is Cronbach's alpha, which can be calculated using the methods that follow.

In the following formulas, reliability of a scale Y is based on adding together k items. The average correlations among items i and j is $\bar{r}_{ij}$ and average covariance among items i and j is $\bar{C}_{ij}$. The variance of item i is σ_i^2. The variance of the scale Y is σ_Y^2.

$$\text{alpha} = r_{kk} = \frac{k}{k-1}\left(1 - \frac{\sum \sigma_i^2}{\sigma_Y^2}\right).$$

Or, if one uses Spearman Brown Prophecy formula, and one (1) replaces average correlation with average covariance, and (2) substitutes average of item variances for the "1" in the denominator, that'll give you alpha too:

Using Spearman Brown Prophecy Formula:

$$r_{kk} = \frac{k\bar{r}_{ij}}{1 + (k-1)\bar{r}_{ij}}.$$

Modified SBPF to yield coefficient alpha:

$$\text{alpha} = r_{kk} = \frac{k\bar{C}_{ij}}{\frac{\sum \sigma_i^2}{k} + (k-1)\bar{C}_{ij}}.$$

Review of these formulas demonstrates that the higher the average correlations among items, the higher the internal consistency reliability. Decisions using this metric will emphasize the selection of items that correlate with other items for inclusion in a measurement. Redundancy is valued with internal consistency reliability.

Given the design considerations of a communimetric tool, one would not expect different items to necessarily correlate with each other. Thus, internal consistency reliability, per se, is not relevant to the evaluation of the individual items of a measure under this theory. You might have items that are related statistically, but you need to include them both because they have different action implications. Or, you might have items that are completely unrelated to each other statistically, but you might still wish to include them in the tool.

An example of the first type of item sets would include depression and anxiety. In planning for mental health treatment it can be important to know both—you have different available treatments for depression and anxiety. From a statistical perspective, these items might be highly correlated and, therefore, might be considered redundant.

Under psychometric theories, you could be justified in dropping one or the other, as your measurement would be relatively unaffected. That would not be the thinking for a communimetric tool. The decision to add or drop an item (or perhaps even combine them) is understood from the value of the relationship to future actions (in this case, treatment planning), not the statistical inter-relationships among items. If you might engage in different actions or interventions based on the presence (or absence) of depression or anxiety, then both need to be included in the tool as separate items.

Although internal consistency reliability is not relevant for the selection of items for a communimetric tool, it can be relevant for determining whether multiple items can be combined to generate dimension scores. For purposes such as monitoring outcomes or change over time, it can be useful to combine multiple items from a communimetric tool into a scale score. Once a decision is made to create scale scores, many of the considerations from psychometric measurement theories become relevant. Cronbach's alpha is an easy and accurate strategy of assessing the degree to which a set of items "hang together" to measure a single construct. Thus, combining items constructed using communimetric theory into a scale requires a minimal level of internal consistency. The general minimum cutoff for this is an alpha of 0.70 or greater as adequate. Very low alphas suggest that the items are unrelated to each other and thus might not be combined into a useful metric. That would not mean, however, that an item that does not fit a dimension score should be eliminated from the tool. The selection of items still should be driven by their individual communication value. It might mean, however, that the non-correlating items would not be used in the creation of a dimension score.

Test–Retest

Often called the stability of a measure, test-retest reliability is calculated by applying the same measurement operation at two different times. The determination of the time difference between T1 and T2 is based on an attempt to remeasure during the same status of the subject (i.e., things haven't changed on relevant constructs) and limiting the effect of practice or memory on the T2 measurement operation (i.e., the person applying the measurement operation does not remember how she or he responded to items at T1). In other words, the time should be close enough to still be measuring the same status, but far enough apart to not simply be a duplication of the prior measurement. This form of reliability is popular for the measure of constructs posited to be stable (i.e., intelligence). This form of reliability is misleading for constructs thought to be unstable or transient (e.g., mood).

Within the communimetric theory of measurement, the concept of test-retest reliability has little or no value. The idea of communimetrics is to obtain information relevant for action and then act based on the information. It is quite relevant to know when you have enough information or the information has stabilized, but you wouldn't conceptualize that as test-retest reliability. The thinking is in reverse. In communimetrics you want to act as soon as the information is actionable, not reassess several weeks later to see whether the information remains stable. Since communimetric tools are designed to assess actionable constructs one hopes that applying the action changes the relevant construct measured by the item. For example, in a new business enterprise, if you have identified an access to commodities needed in your production analysis, you want to address it, not make sure that need remains stable. The relevant stability question then predates the application of the communimetric measurement operation. Therefore, test-retest reliability of the measure is not relevant. You want to identify addressable needs, which by definition should not be stable in the face of action. Whether or not they are stable in the face of no action is not particularly interesting. You would never apply the measurement process in the absence of the human service context.

Inter-rater

This form of reliability is an absolute requirement of a communimetric tool. It is impossible to pursue a measurement strategy based on communication that does not consider the accuracy of that communication. The concept of inter-rater reliability in communimetric tools is whether or not two different raters are using the language of the tool in comparable ways.

There are many outstanding articles and books on the subject of reliability and there are many useful options to consider for determining the inter-rater reliability of a measure. The two most common are kappa and intraclass correlation coefficients (ICC).

Kappa is a good approach when the scale of the measure is categorical. The reliability of present/absent ratings are best estimated using kappa as is any measurement strategy that involves assigning observations to categories.

ICC is the recommended approach when the rating scale can be assumed to at least be ordinal. In other words, is there any meaningful ordering to the possible ratings. If so, then it is possible to be close but still wrong. With kappa, the rater is either wrong or right (excepting weighted kappas, of course, which function more like an ICC). With ICC the rater is given some credit for being close. So if the recommended rating is a 2 and the rater selected 1, it is given more credit than if he or she selected 0. Given the design of action levels on most communimetric tools, an ICC is the recommended strategy for estimating inter-rater reliability.

Intraclass Correlation Computation Procedure: ICC(3,1)
Inter-rater reliability is estimated using formula for ICC(3,1), two-way mixed model case, as described in Shrout and Fleiss (1979). Specifically, for each person who completes a set of vignette ratings, a matrix of rater and key ratings are generated for each target. This formula is applied to the values in this matrix. For example, consider the following 2×8 matrix:

The ICC(3,1) formula estimates the correlation between Rater scores and Key (i.e., correct) scores. To calculate ICC(3,1), one must estimate Between Target Mean Square (BMS) and Error Mean Square (EMS). These statistics require calculations of row, column, and total sums, and a number of sums of squared values. For example:

Before calculating BMS and EMS, we calculate 4 "basic ratios," that include various kinds of sums of squared sums, denoted: $[X]$, $[J]$, $[T]$, and $[C]$.

$$[X]=\sum_{i=1}^{n}\sum_{j=1}^{2}X_{ij}^{2}=3^{2}+2^{2}+1^{2}+1^{2}+\cdots+2^{2}+2^{2}+1^{2}+1^{2}=62$$

$$[J]=\frac{\sum_{j=1}^{2}\left(\sum_{i=1}^{n}X_{ij}\right)^{2}}{n}=\frac{13^{2}+15^{2}}{8}=49.25$$

$$[T]=\frac{\sum_{i=1}^{n}\left(\sum_{j=1}^{2}X_{ij}\right)^{2}}{2}=\frac{5^{2}+2^{2}+1^{2}+5^{2}+6^{2}+3^{2}+4^{2}+2^{2}}{2}=\frac{120}{2}=60$$

$$[C]=\frac{\sum_{i=1}^{n}\left(\sum_{j=1}^{2}X_{ij}\right)^{2}}{2n}=\frac{(3+2+1+1+\cdots+2+2+1+1)^{2}}{2(8)}=\frac{28^{2}}{16}=49.$$

The BMS is calculated as follows (with example):

$$\text{BMS}=[T]-[C]=60-49=11.$$

The EMS is calculated as follows (with example):

$$\text{EMS}=[X]-[J]-[T]+[C]=62-49.25-60+49=1.75.$$

The final calculation, is based on BMS and EMS, as follows (with example):

$$\text{ICC}(3,1)=\frac{\text{BMS}-\text{EMS}}{\text{BMS}+\text{EMS}}=\frac{11-1.75}{11+1.75}=0.7255\approx 0.72.$$

The answer should be rounded to 2 decimals, for presentation purposes.

Estimation via SPSS

If evaluated via SPSS, the data are entered as above (two columns, "key" and "rater"), and the following syntax will generate the correct answer (syntax and output follow). The correct answer is found in the "single measures" line.

```
RELIABILITY
/VARIABLES=rater key
/FORMAT=NOLABELS
/SCALE(ALPHA)=ALL/MODEL=ALPHA
/ICC=MODEL(MIXED) TYPE(CONSISTENCY) CIN=95 TESTVAL=0.
```

Audit Reliability

Of course, the real test of the reliability of any measurement operation is whether it can be accurately applied in the settings where it is actually used. For communimetric tools, this is reliability within human service enterprises. A form of reliability that is both feasible and desirable with communimetric measures is audit reliability—a comparison of a prospectively completed measure to the same measure completed retrospectively using different information sources covering a comparable period of time.

The concept of audit reliability is important at several levels. First, it is important to document the field reliability of a measure if you want to use the information from that measure to draw meaningful conclusions. Applications of the tool that follow the scientific method require good reliability. Audit reliability is as good or better an estimate compared with any other form of inter-rater reliability in the field. Of course, one could have two people serve the same client at the same time and fill out the tool independently, but this is both time consuming and expensive and might very well change the nature of the interaction between the client and providers. It is hard to imagine that the client could maintain precisely the same approach both times. Alternatively, one could videotape an assessment interview and have someone independently complete the tool. Of course, videotaping requires consent and may again change the nature of the communication. Two people could sit in on the same assessment and one could complete the tool with the client and the other on their own, but it is unclear what a high correlation between the two raters would mean under these circumstances. Therefore, most alternative methods are expensive and intrusive and are very unlikely to ever happen outside of a research project. Audit reliability, on the other hand, can be implemented as a business practice.

In an audit method, a random sample of cases is taken. It might be stratified by agency or assessor depending on whether you would like to generalize the reliability findings to specific strata (i.e., groups). If you want to talk about the reliability of individuals, then you should stratify your sample on those individuals to ensure all are equally and effectively represented. Likewise, if you want to report on the reliability of programs or agencies, the same logic holds. Random samples of cases should be drawn from any group to which you would like to ascribe reliability.

Once the cases have been sampled, a trained assessor would complete the tool independently from the one completed prospectively in the process of providing assistance. Other documentation, such as written summaries or treatment plans, are used to provide the information to allow the auditor to complete the tool. Once the audit has been completed, you compare the auditor ratings to the original ratings using the ICC described in the preceding section. There are several published examples of audits using communimetric tools in behavioral health (Anderson, Lyons, Giles, Price, & Estle, 2003; Lyons, Rawal, Yeh, Leon, & Tracy, 2001). In both of these reports, the communimetric tool was reliable in the field. Anderson et al. report describes item level reliability as well. Item reliability was quite high for most items.

The ability to audit depends in large part on the availability of adequate records concurrent with the prospective completion of the tool. Those records must contain the type of information necessary to complete the tool. This requirement has not been a problem in health care and behavioral health, as medical charts often contain written summaries that cover the same topical areas as the communimetric measure. Given that that actual process of delivering care is used to design the measure, it should not be particularly surprising that the written assessments and communimetric tools have overlapping content.

The absence of reliability during an audit can come from at least three possible sources and a failure to find reliability should be understood within this context. First, it may be a characteristic of the measure. It is possible that the field reliability of an item or a tool is insufficient. This conclusion suggests that refinement of the tool or training process should be undertaken. Second, it may reflect the reliability of the auditor. Because of this possible conclusion, it is useful to use multiple auditors to compare the relative reliability between them as a possible interpretation. Third, it is possible that the available records did not contain sufficient information to allow for the reliable completion of the tool. This conclusion is a quality improvement finding relevant for the improvement of the target agency, program, or assessors records.

Validity

The validity of a measure is the degree to which the number(s) accurately reflects the construct and the level of the construct the measure is attempting to describe. Or, is the measure assessing what it purports to measure? While this question may sound simple, it unfolds as an onion into a variety of rather complex considerations. Psychometric theorists have spent a great deal of time on the concept of validity. Traditional views of measurement have established a number of different ways in which to understand this phenomenon.

Face validity is the degree to which a measure "looks like" what it purports to measure. If a naïve person picks up a copy of the measure and reads it, he or she could guess what it is trying to measure. Face validity was originally seen as a way to ensure participation of respondents. People tend to prefer to answer questions that seem relevant. Face validity is thought to be far more important in communimetric and clinimetric conceptualization of the measurement process than in psychometric approaches. Feinstein (1986) places face validity as the most important consideration and uses this difference in priority to highlight the distinction between clinimetric and psychometrics. In clinimetrics, however, face validity is with the physician or other health professional. It is considered essential to the overall validity of the measure that the physician understand the relationship of the measure to the clinical status of the patient. Face validity is a necessary but insufficient validity consideration for a communimetric tool.

Traditionally, concern regarding face validity has been expressed by some psychometricians (e.g., Anastasi, 1968; Nunally, 1976). There are circumstances in which respondents might not be honest if they fully understand what you are asking. The MMPI has validity scales embedded in an attempt to detect lying and faking bad. So, when concerns about hypothesis guessing are paramount, face validity can be seen as a problem (If the respondent knows what you are trying to measure, he or she might actively choose to misrepresent their true response.)

In most cases, people seeking help are straightforward and forthright about attempting to accurately communicate their needs. However, there can be circumstances in human service enterprises in which clients might be less than forthcoming about information relevant to planning for their needs. In general, these circumstances involve the client seeking some benefit to which it is feared that he or she is not entitled. Workmen's compensation is an unfortunate, but common, example, but so can be housing services, public welfare, and in some circumstances behavioral health treatment. In these circumstances a subset of people might be tempted to lie in order to get something they are otherwise not entitled to receive. Alternatively, there are circumstances in which errors or omission (not being open about actual needs) is the greater problem, as a subset of individuals' attempts to avoid something they do not wish to receive.

It has been my experience that these concerns are very real. People do sometime lie and mislead. However, the vast majority of people seeking to engage human services enterprises are simply seeking help and present their needs as accurately as they know how. Therefore, it is bad policy to structure the measurement process on the premise that the client will be less than fully honest. Creating universal policies based on exceptions is generally bad policy (Lyons, 2004). However, creating flexibility to address deviations from the norm is good policy. That is why communimetric measures use information-integration strategies. By combining information from various sources to establish the level of need, it is possible to still work with the client who is struggling with his or her own openness or honesty. Consequently, despite the threat that might come from the respondent knowing the meaning of a measure to the respondent, the value of this knowledge for creating a collaborative, open, and direct helping environment far outweighs the disadvantages that might arise from face validity. The opportunity to engage in constitutive communication (i.e., meaning making) is dramatically enhanced by the face validity of the tool.

Content validity is related to face validity in that it focuses on how the items in the measure look, but in this form of validity the focus is more on theoretical and statistical considerations rather than on issues of user-interface. Content validity is the focus of the item analysis in classical test theory and item fit statistics in item response theory. Content validity is a core construct for both clinimetric and communimetric theories of measurement. Content validity sometimes works differently with psychometric theories. These approaches emphasize statistical characteristics of items; however, when items are found to form factor structures, the content of related items is often used to name the factor.

Construct validity is the broadest and most complex conceptualization of validity from traditional measurement perspectives. This form of validity seeks to document that the measure is, in fact, assessing the construct(s) it is purporting to measure.

Does a measure of depression actually measure the phenomenon of depression? Does a job skills survey actually measure the skills a person can apply in a work setting? Effectively addressing these questions can be quite complex, and many methodological approaches have been identified to gauge a measure's construct validity.

Construct validity is demonstrated through an ensemble of different types of comparisons. These component analyses are often given names as different forms of validity. For example, concurrent validity describes whether a measure is related to other measures that purport to measure the same things. Divergent validity is used to describe whether the measure is not related to things to which it should not be related or is negatively related to things that are thought to be opposite. Predictive validity refers to whether a measure can predict events and states in the future that are relevant to the construct measured. There are a wide variety of methods and statistical procedures that can be used to build a case for construct validity. It is generally accepted that no single study can be used to fully establish the construct validity of a measure (Anastasi, 1968; Nunally, 1976).

While all of the traditional forms of validity are important considerations for a communimetric measure to varying degrees, the concept of validity must be expanded in light of the purposed communication role of these measures. The additional form of validity is the value of the tool in the human service enterprise—the utility validity.

Utility Validity

The concept that a measure is useful within a service delivery system is not new. Most measurement experts who have attempted to implement a measure within a human service enterprise will state that it is important that the measure at least be easy to use if not actually immediately and directly useful. They also may emphasize the importance of predictive validity as an indicator of usefulness. However, from the perspective of communimetrics the utility of the measure in the service delivery operations is the single most important validity consideration and, therefore, requires a more complete conceptualization of exactly how this form of validity is understood and assessed.

One might make an argument that utility validity is some combination of face and content validity, and therefore, is nothing new. In other words, if the measure looks like what it should look like to its users and contains the information relevant to its purpose, then it is de facto useful. But that argument reflects an incomplete understanding of the concept of utility in the communimetric theory of measurement.

As discussed in earlier chapters, the consideration of measurement in service delivery is a fundamentally different enterprise than measurement during research and evaluation. A significant difference results from the fact that research and evaluation efforts are generally required to use informed consent, confidentiality, and anonymity to help ensure the veridicality (truthfulness or accuracy; that is, validity) of the measures. That respondents do not have any known agenda in choosing their responses is fundamental to the research enterprise. The vast majority of traditional measurement work has been done within this context of informed consent. Therefore, if the development and testing of most other measures are subject to the constraint that measurement occurred in a neutral environment in which scores on the measure had absolutely no impact on what happened next. The measures are valid in the context of informed consent, confidentiality, and anonymity. As Cook (2007) states, "all performance indicators are subject to corruption." There is no perfect measure; they are all flawed. When you use measures outside the parameters of the context of research and evaluation, they are subject to these biases. Any measure can be faked by the motivated respondent.

As a result, in the absence of informed consent, confidentiality, and anonymity—which are challenging if not impossible in service delivery settings, particularly when considering the context of performance-based contracting (e.g., pay for performance)—what options do we have to help ensure that rating scales are valid? In fact, there are a number of things we can do to help ensure such accuracy. These steps are the methodological foundation of creating or enhancing utility validity.

Relevance to the work

To the degree that the measurement process is the same as the work, respondents are more motivated to complete them fully and accurately. When a measure informs the planning process with the individual recipient, it becomes clearly unethical to falsely assess and falsely serve. If supervisors are taught to work with direct service staff using the measurement tools, this involvement increases the importance of the tool to the work, and therefore enhances accuracy. Most traditional measurement approaches function as exclusively research and evaluation measures, which are not designed to be relevant to service planning. They simply document aspects of that process and are reported out, often anonymously. This guarantees that some people will see them only as an unnecessary reporting burden and not something in which accuracy is a paramount consideration (or, sometimes even a consideration at all). As a counterpoint, one could also make the counterargument that by making a measure relevant to the work it increases the motivation to falsely represent the data. That concern would be operable in circumstances in which the respondent was concerned about the implications of accurate measurement (e.g., change in payment or scrutiny). This type of faking of results is less of a concern if the relevant measure is used in a culture of openness, transparency, and accountability.

Transparency

A very important strategy for ensuring the reliability and validity of an application is to make it as transparent as possible. Since communimetric measurement is an information-integration strategy it can be completed without the individual who is described by the measurement. Although this is sometimes a necessary consequence of a particular application (i.e., file review), it is not the recommended approach. In fact, ensuring that the individual described has seen the description and understand the implications of the results of applying the measurement approach is a far more desirable situation. This is the primary level of transparency. The individual and the person completing the measurement share the results of the measure openly.

I strongly recommend using structured communimetric tools in supervision. It provides the supervisor with information on how the supervisee conceptualizes his or her work. Communimetric measures are designed to communicate, so it is important to use them in that way. Openness encourages honesty and accuracy.

A validity consideration from psychometrics, face validity, is important for this strategy. Face validity refers to the degree to which the measure looks like what it is supposed to be measuring "on the face of it." In other words, if everyone looks at a measure and says it makes sense, then it has face validity. While face validity is generally thought of as a less important form of validity in psychometrics, it is essential in communimetrics. Measuring a construct using indirect or obtuse questions or subtly trying to assess something that the respondent may not be aware of is not the goal of communimetrics. It is exactly the opposite. The philosophy is, "What do you need to know, and how can I help you know it?" Communication is the foundation of relationships; trust is required for effective communication. Trust must be explicit in the measurement process to reinforce the actual use of the measurement approach. Therefore, face validity is a requirement of a communimetric measure. And the same concept of face validity should extend to all applications of the measure.

To the degree that multiple parties witness the completion of a measure and all understand its implications and how it is used, accuracy will be enhanced. Measurement processes that are shared across partners in the intervention planning process are optimal. For example, in child behavioral health, use of child-family team models that pull together everyone who is involved in the life of a particular child, have been used to ensure that assessments achieve consensus and all relevant parties have input into considerations. Measures completed by one person in isolation are much more likely to be fraught with problems with accuracy than measures that are widely and openly shared. For this reason, the communication value of a measure is paramount. To ensure transparency, all parties in a process should be able to understand the meaning and implications of a measure so that checks and balances can be applied. In some cases, meeting this objective may require training for some parties who will not have to complete the measure, but still must know what it means.

Multiple purposes

It is not uncommon for measures to be required by states or other funding entities for performance monitoring and/or management purposes. These applications are often experienced as unfunded mandates by human service providers.

In these situations, measures simply represent a documentation/reporting function required to get paid (or stay out of trouble). This type of application generates a couple of significant challenges. First, providers naturally resent the time and expense of completing the tool. Second, there is no value to the provider except to ensure payment. Therefore, the contingencies of these measures place natural pressure on respondents to attempt to report what they believe the funding source would like to see. This can be an enormous problem in many performance monitoring projects that have only this narrow focus. That's why some people don't trust DSM-IV diagnoses in Medicaid data sets—they were simply generated to ensure payment. It also is the reason for the failure of Indiana's application of standard assessment tool prior to their decision to implement the CANS. The initial measure served only to ensure funding and became a burden on providers while providing no meaningful information to the state. In fact, providers had a very cynical name for the process of completing the measure annually—"the dash for cash." That culture was one of the primary reasons Indiana decided to shift to the CANS and a Total Clinical Outcome Management (TCOM) strategy (Lyons, 2004). TCOM is the larger conceptual approach of which CANS is a component. As described in Chap. 3, an essential premise of this strategy is that if providers must complete a measure anyway, why not make it useful to them for the multiple purposes for which a measure can be used?

When one measure has multiple applications, it enhances its reliability and validity because the value of the information in the measure is increased by these uses. The more information matters to more different people, the more likely it is that everyone will participate in ensuring that the information is accurate and useful.

This method of ensuring reliability and validity is actually in counterpoint to how research measures are generally designed. In research, measurement is kept confidentially, uses are specifically limited, and information is not shared. The confidentiality with which information is kept is thought to be central to maintaining the integrity of the research and helping individuals feel like they can be honest and open in answering the questions that are the inputs of the measurement process.

In human service settings, an entirely different set of contingencies operate. Often, individuals and families become tired of answering the same questions again and again at different stages of the service delivery process. Further, when different people want different information they are all loaded into assessment processes. The requirement of obtaining all the required information becomes a burden and the quality of the information suffers as a result.

Correspondence to sociopolitical considerations

In some circles, even mention of sociopolitical considerations in the development and use of a measurement strategy would be scientific heresy. Science is the enterprise of elucidating the truth, and political considerations have no place in such an enterprise. Unfortunately, in field applications political considerations can have major implications for the success of the implementation process. Failure to attend to critical people and processes can sabotage the implementation of even a highly useful measure. One person in a position of relative power with a significant ego or issues of personal control can block many things from happening.

As discussed in Chap. 1, the epistemology of measurement in human service enterprises requires attention to sociopolitical processes. This challenge draws comparisons with relativist philosophy of science. If sociopolitical processes can influence measurement processes, then isn't this proof that they are not measuring some objective reality as proposed by the logical positivists, but rather some social construction consistent with the beliefs of the relativists? As discussed in Chap. 1, that is not necessarily true. By adopting a realist perspective, it is possible to understand that the view of objective reality might be influenced by social forces but not necessarily defined. Much like looking out the window of a moving train, perhaps sometime you need to adjust your view to see the same thing that you observed before. Just because you are moving does not necessarily mean that what you are observing is changing. What changes is the perspective from which you observe.

Communication is a function of language and language is influenced by culture. Language is in a constant state of flux. Over time, different words are used to describe the same things. The same word begins to mean different things overtime. This does not change the nature of the dialog, just the words that are used in that dialog.

Indicators of Utility Validity

There are a number of ways to assess the utility validity of a measure, including the following:

Respondent satisfaction

This indicator if the degree to which respondents who complete the measure are satisfied that the measure supports their work. The components of this concept might include the degree to which they understand the measure, feel comfortable completing it, and use it to guide decisions.

Relationship to subsequent action

An unobtrusive measure of utility validity is the relationship between assessed characteristics on a measure and the subsequent actions taken following the measurement process. The intended relationship to subsequent action is the principal characteristic of a communimetric tool. Therefore, assessing whether or not a correspondence exists can be used as an indicator of utility validity.

Use penetration

It can be difficult to fully implement the use of any structured measurement/assessment process in a human service context. Thus the completeness of an implementation is a very useful indicator of utility validity. The easiest use penetration metric is:

$$\text{Use penetration} = \frac{\text{Number of times the measure completed}}{\text{Number of times the measure should be completed}}.$$

The denominator being the number of instances in which the measure would be completed if always used when indicated by the protocol. The closer to 100%, the better the utility validity.

The parallel of use penetration in scientific methods would be response rate. The concept of response rate is the percent of potential respondents who participate in a study. There is no real statistical difference between response rate and use penetration. The difference is conceptual. There is no reason to sample use penetration. It should be monitored as an ongoing evaluation of the validity of the measure. It should be a population-based statistic, not one based on a sample. Commonly the greatest challenge to calculating use penetration is determining the denominator. You need an independent source of information about when a specific tool should be used.

Use penetration is an indicator of utility validity only when the effort is to implement a communimetric tool uniformly throughout a system. Of course, if you are using the tool on an ad hoc basis and not throughout a system, then use penetration is not important and may not even be able to be calculated.

Table 4.1 presents the use penetration of the Child and Adolescent Needs and Strengths (CANS) tool in the child welfare system in the central region of Tennessee. In this system, child protective services and case workers are to team to complete the CANS in time for the child and family team meeting approximately 7 days after custody of a child is taken.

Impact evaluation

Ultimately, a communimetric tool anticipates having an impact on practice. Thus, the very fact of implementing the measurement strategy is expected to potentially change in the performance of the system in which it is implemented. Communimetrics value the functioning of the system. A tool designed to enhance communication efficiency

Table 4.1 Use Penetration of the CANS in Central Tennessee Child Welfare System

	July, 2007			August, 2007			September, 2007			October, 2007		
Region	CANS	Children	%	CANS	Childrens	%	CANS	Children	%	CANS	Children	%
Davidson	14	14	100	17	20	85	17	18	94	25	36	69
Hamilton	16	16	100	12	17	74	12	12	100	19	20	95
Midcumberland	31	69	45	11	58	19	38	82	48	31	68	54
South Central	17	19	89	37	38	97	25	30	83	37	37	100
South East	13	13	100	29	29	-100	26	26	100	27	27	100
Uppercumberland	14	20	70	15	21	71	20	25	80	24	27	89
Total	105	151	70	123	185	66	138	193	72	163	215	76

and accuracy should have an impact at minimum on the quality of communication in the system. In fact, in discussing the implementation of people using communimetric tools they often comment on the transformation impact of using the tool itself.

While the tool should support improved communication, its impact should be much broader than that at least in most circumstances. The proposed impact, of course, will vary with the nature and use of the tool. The implementation of an enterprise development tool should result in improved business outcomes for the participating enterprises. A behavioral health assessment tool that is used primarily for decision support should result in improved concordance and ultimately better functional outcomes for targeted programs/interventions. A biopsychosocial assessment in primary care setting might result in more integrated care and a reduction in excessive health service utilization.

Given the potential diversity of impacts it is impossible to inventory all possibilities. Therefore, I can only make general recommendations about approaching impact analysis. As with any research, the first step is to ask the question. In this case, the question is, Where would we anticipate seeing an impact of implementing a specific tool? Start with the affected parties (e.g., people completing the tool and people being described with the tool) and move to higher levels of aggregation from there (e.g., individual programs, systems, or markets or jurisdictions).

The field of cliometrics offers some potential insights into how to approach impact analysis in some settings. Cliometrics is the use of archival quantitative economic data to study historically relevant questions (Fogel, 1964; Lyons, Cain, & Williamson, 2008). Robert Fogel and Douglas North won the Nobel Prize in Economics in 1993 for their work developing cliometrics. In 2006, a new journal, *Cliometrica—Journal of Historical Economics and Econometric History,* was launched.

Decision Validity

Decision validity is a form of validity that applies to the decision support applications for communimetric tools. This validity combines features of both construct and predictive validity from traditional conceptualizations (e.g., Anastasi, 1968). However, in human service enterprises, assessing the quality of decisions is sufficiently unique from a conceptual and methodological perspective to speak of unique validity considerations for these applications.

As described in Chap. 3, there are essentially two methods for using decision support applications for communimetric tools—eligibility and quality improvement. These two approaches have overlapping but at time different validity considerations.

For both models, concordance is a first level validity indicator. Is the recommendation of the tool consistent with what actually has been decided? For example, using the CANS to support decisions regarding residential treatment in child welfare in Illinois, Chor et al. (2008) recently reported 385 out of 466 (82.6%) decisions to place a child/youth in residential treatment were concordant with the CANS recommendation. This percent is a high enough rate to suggest that the recommendation of the tool is consistent enough with standard practice. Concordance rates are similar to reliabilities in their interpretation. Below 60% should be viewed as problematic; between 60 and 70% is marginal; above 70% is adequate; above 80% is good; above 90% is excellent.

Outcome differences are the most important validity indicator for all decision support models. Outcome differences; however, are not always straightforward as they require a 2 × 2 contingency table of findings to be fully interpretable, as described in Table 4.2. People recommended for the program/intervention that should have reliably better outcomes from that program/intervention than do people receive the program/intervention but are not recommended (cell D vs. cell C). And people who fail to receive the recommended program/intervention should have worse outcomes than those who are not recommended and do receive the program/intervention (cell B vs. cell C). And, of course, people who receive the recommended program/intervention should have better outcomes than those who are recommended but do not receive (cell D vs. cell B).

A variety of circumstances make actually completing this type of validity study quite challenging. First, factors relating to the actual decisions about both the recommendation for the program/intervention and the actual reception may be correlated with outcomes. Membership in these cells is never randomly assigned. Therefore, baseline differences will exist making change analysis challenging. Since the decision models are correlated with status at admission, covariate and percent change models may not make sense as strategies to provide some methodological control.

Second, sometimes it is difficult to follow along with people who do not receive a program/intervention to monitor their status in the absence of interventions. Often, information is available at the time of the recommendation and decision about actual receipt, but only those who receive the program/intervention are then followed, leaving no outcome data in cells A and B. Cell A is not necessary to complete the analyses, but cell B provides important information about the relative value of failure to intervene (e.g., the opportunity cost of not receiving a recommended program/intervention).

One option to address the nonequivalence of groups is propensity analysis (D'Agostino, 1998; Rosenbaum & Rubin, 1983). This statistical approach allows the matching of groups on a number of potential confounding factors in order to achieve reasonably comparable groups. Figure 4.1 provides a propensity validation of a model of decision support for psychiatric hospitalization

Table 4.2 Decision analysis framework for understanding outcomes by recommendation versus receipt of an intervention or program

	Tool Does Not Recommend Program/Intervention	Tool Recommends Program/Intervention
Person does not receive program/intervention	(A) Not recommended, does not receive	(B) Recommended, does not receive
Person does receive program/intervention	(C) Not recommended but receives	(D) Recommended and receives

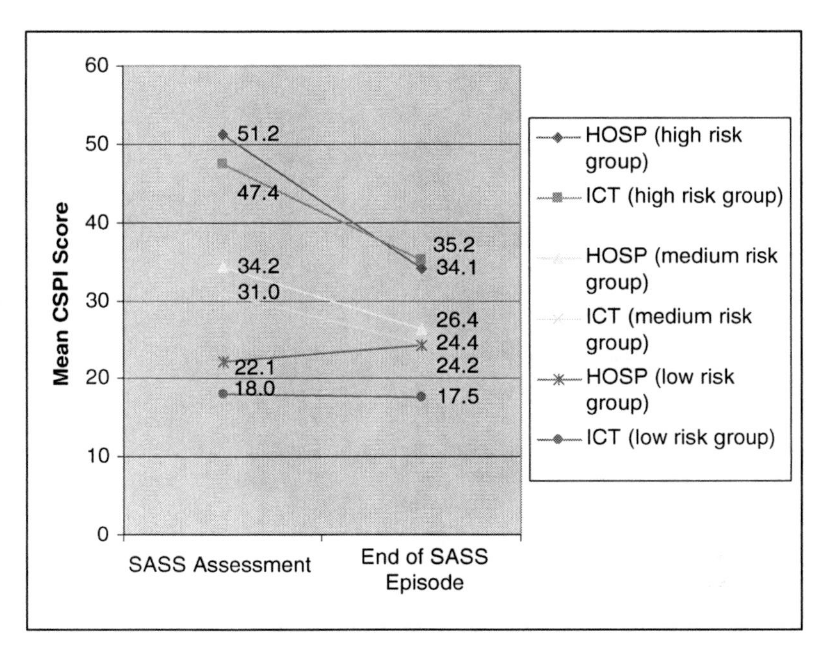

Fig. 4.1 A propensity analysis of children and youth served in a mobile crisis program in Illinois

of children and youth. This program screened for the need for psychiatric hospitalization. They use one of the original communimetric tools the Childhood Severity of Psychiatric Illness (CSPI; Lyons, Mintzer, Kisiel, & Shallcross, 1998). This tool has a demonstrated relationship to decisions about the use of psychiatric hospitalization (He, Lyons, & Heinemann, 2004; Snowden, Leon, Bryant, & Lyons, 2007).

A second alternative to manage unequal groups is to use repeated measure or growth curve analyses (Duncan, Duncan, Strycker, Li, & Alpert, 1999). Figure 4.2 plots the level of Emotional/Behavioral needs from the CANS for children/youth recommended for residential treatment who were placed (Concordant) to those not recommended, but who were still placed in residential treatment (Discordant). Figure 4.2 provides the same information for Risk Behaviors. Clearly, the concordant group stated out with a higher level of needs than the discordant group but got better. The discordant group got worse on Emotional/Behavior needs and somewhat better on Risk Behaviors. Review of this figure provides validity support for the CANS decision model. You don't need to statistically match the two groups and, in fact, it might be misleading to do so since they are so different on the key outcome anyway. With growth curve analysis you can compare the slopes and intercepts for the growth curves as relative outcomes. You would propose steeper slopes for the concordant groups.

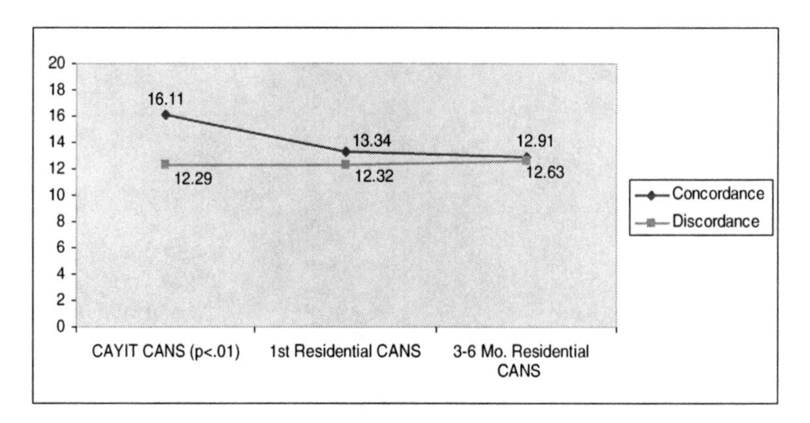

Fig. 4.2 The level of Emotional/Behavioral needs from the CANS for children/youth recommended for residential treatment who were placed (Concordant) to those not recommended, but who were still placed in residential treatment (Discordant)

Enhancing the Reliability and Validity Through Training

Since communimetric tools are different than most other measurement strategies in both their design and use, it is almost always necessary to train new users of these measures in their proper application. In general, training requires the explanation of the approach, practice on applying the measurement approach to examples, and certification that the trainee is able to use the measure reliably on a test example. Certification of reliability is quite important to this approach in that you really do not want people completing the tool who are using it incorrectly. When others see a completed measure that is patently wrong, it damages trust in the tool or in the process. Since effective communication is based on trust, certification of reliability prior to permission to use a tool is an effective means of building trust. Maintaining ongoing reliability further reinforces that trust.

In many of the current applications of communimetric tools, we require annual recertification. In other words, users must complete a test case vignette and achieve a sufficient level of reliability in order to continue to use the tool. Recertification processes are helpful at several levels. First, the fact that recertification exists, lets all users know that reliability is an ongoing priority to the measurement process. This notice functions much like the sign on the door advertising a burglar alarm. It simply notifies people to take the training and use seriously. Second, recertification helps ensure against reliability decay (Bakeman & Gottman, 1997). It is a widely held belief that without periodically checking in on the reliability of a measurement process, the reliability of that process declines with time. Checking in annually is not particularly time consuming and appears to provide some protections. For example, Table 4.3 presents the average recertification reliability from 2004 to 2007 on two related tools. This table contains the average annual intraclass correlation coefficients for recertification on the CANS. In addition, the range of reliability

Table 4.3 Annual Recertification Statistics for the System of Care—Foster Care Stabilization Program's Use of the Child and Adolescent Needs and Strengths (CANS) Tool

Year	# Staff Tested	# Passed on First Try	Average Reliability
2004	255	139	0.68
2005	189	133	0.73
2006	190	189	0.87
2007	230	223	0.78

scores and the percent of recertifiers who did not pass on the first attempt is provided. Review of these data support the ongoing improvement in reliability during the process of annual recertification. The data from 2006 is a bit of an outlier in that the average reliability was very high, in part, due to a stable work force. The year 2007 witnessed an expansion of the number of SOC staff and a subsequent decline in recertification average reliability as a number of these individuals were being recertified for the first time.

Field audit

Another strategy to ensure reliability and validity in the actual practice is to utilize field audits. In other words, treat the information collected about the people served with the same seriousness and oversight used to monitor the financial operations. One of the major advantages of the use of an information integration strategy in the design of the measure is that it supports audit methodologies. Since communimetric measures can be completed using information from any number of sources, it can easily be audited when completed prospectively as a part of a human services delivery system.

In the first published audit of a communimetric measure, Anderson et al. (2003) demonstrated that for most individual items on the CANS, the audit reliability was greater than 0.70 using an intraclass correlation coefficient. In this project, audit reliability was defined as the comparison of ratings of clinicians completing the CANS prospectively in their work with children and youth to research assistants, trained in the reliable use of the CANS using clinical records independently. The reliability of two research assistants using precisely the same information to make ratings was quite high for nearly every item of the measure.

Enhancing the Reliability and Validity Through Use

The single best strategy to ensure that a measure is used with reliability and validity is to make sure that it is, in fact, fully utilized. Communimetric tools exist to communicate. If they are completed and placed in a database or file, they will not serve their primary purpose and, in all likelihood, the reliability with which they are completed may decline along with the validity of the information contained in the measure. The same problems exist for communimetrics tools. Nonuse can be a significant threat to reliability and, hence, validity of a measure used in an applied setting. The difference between the two approaches is that the ways in which a communimetric can be utilized within the human service enterprise setting.

The levels of use can be described using the following three categories:

- Form—something I have to fill out because someone told me to do it
- Tool—something that helps me in my work
- Framework—this is my work

Unfortunately, most measurement processes in human services are not integrated into the work, and people who complete them often experience them as paperwork that is required but not relevant. This problem is a significant barrier to the reliability and validity of applied measurement.

The design of communimetric tools allow them to be used as both tools and frameworks. However, the design itself is generally insufficient to get most people who have already developed beliefs and behaviors around forms to embrace this paradigm shift. A number of strategies can be used to enhance the likelihood that people completing communimetric measures recognize their potential as tools or even as a framework (Lyons, 2004; Lyons & Weiner, 2009).

The Convergence of Communimetric and Psychometric Approaches with the Use of Aggregate Item Analyses

Communimetric measures are designed to be useful at the individual level without scoring or through using Bayesian logic models (e.g., the decision algorithms discussed in this text) to make recommendations for decision support applications. However, they also claim to be useful for understanding information at the program and system level. Of course the least sophisticated approach to aggregate analyses is to report frequencies of item ratings of proportions or percents of populations. These types of analyses require no assumptions to permit their valid application in any setting in which a communimetric measure is used. However, most program and system level analyses require a more sophisticated approach to data analyses. To achieve the goals of many of these analyses, dimension scores across multiple items become desirable. Single items can burden an analysis that seeks to make broad generalizations about a program or system. As soon as one seeks to use scale or dimension scores coming from a communimetric measure, the assumptions, considerations, and strategies that have arisen from psychometric theories become critical. Statistical analysis of aggregated data is where the communimetric and psychometric theories converge. Or, perhaps it is more accurate to say that it is in these analyses that communimetric measurement becomes subsumed under the rules of psychometric theories.

We have subjected a number of communimetric tools to psychometric analysis and it appears that generally the dimension scores generated from a communimetric tool have solid psychometric properties from both a classical test and item response theory perspectives. Many other resources are available to the interested reader regarding the specific statistical analyses used in psychometrics. However, a number of these approaches will be used to study dimension scores in the chapters that detail examples of communimetric measures.

Comparing Versions

Because of features in the design process, communimetric tools are often modified somewhat across different jurisdictions. They can introduce challenges when there is interest in comparing experiences across these jurisdictions. There is value in standardization. There is also value in tailoring to accommodate local variations. To balance this tension by optimizing the benchmarking value of communimetric tools while maintaining their design flexibility for local implementations, a few rules have been established.

An item is an item is an item regardless of version. Once an item is created and named, the effort is to maintain the integrity of this item. The item Danger to Others is the same item in all versions of the CANS. A rating of 0 indicates no evidence; a 1 indicates notable history or suspicion, a rating of 2 indicates recent violence or notable threat, and a rating of 3 is acute, today. If you have this item on your version, this is what it means. This item is designed from a behavioral health perspective, as danger to other people is a risk behavior that leads to elevated levels of care in mental health. There are some versions of the CANS that consider violence in different ways. Some versions used in child welfare have an item named Violence, which has a different set of anchors that extends the time frames for ratings of 2 and 3. Therefore, the rule is that if you change the item fundamentally, you need to label it with a different name.

Try to use as many of the same items as possible. Establishing a core set of items within a field is useful. For example, there are about 30 items on the CANS that almost everyone uses. They have strong reliability, validity, and utility and there is no good reason to change them. Adding new items makes sense if either the construct is not currently included or if it is too embedded in another item and needs to be separated for intervention planning purposes. These later situations are the most complicated for efforts to combined findings across versions.

An example from the CANS is helpful to clarify the optimal strategy. The original versions of the CANS had a single School Functioning item. Early applications were in acute care and residential treatment settings. Knowing whether or not the child/youth was having any problems in school was sufficient. As more (and different) people became involved in using the CANS, the need for a finer-grained communication was identified. The second version of the CANS-MH took the single school item and divided it into three items: School Behavior (How does the child/youth act while in school?), School Attendance (Does the child go to school consistently?), and School Achievement (What is his or her academic functioning?). All items use standard action levels, so if you wanted to return to the original single rating you would simply take the highest rating among the three new, finer-grained ratings. A child with a 2 on School Behavior would have a 2 on School Functioning. But a child with a 2 on School Attendance would also have a 2 on School Functioning. With this design it is also possible to go to a higher level of abstraction on any domain of information. However, it is not possible to take the School Functioning rating and extrapolate into the three finer-grained school items.

Severity and Complexity

Traditional measurement has focused on locating individuals on latent traits—unseen constructs. When applied to needs, this approach leads to the use of dimension scores to assess severity. However, the severity or intensity of a dimension is only one way to conceptualize how a person presents to human service enterprises. A second characteristic is the complexity of need(s).

Severity is the noun tense of the word *severe*. While severe has multiple connotations, one meaning is "to a great degree" (Merriam-Webster On-Line Dictionary, 2008). Severity connotes a high degree of a specific need. Complexity is defined as "the quality or state of being complex." Complex also has multiple meaning and one is "a sum of factors (as symptoms) characterizing a disease or condition." Perhaps an even more relevant definition is, "a whole made up of complicated or interrelated parts." Complexity connotes a lot of different but related things going on simultaneously. While severity and complexity are related, they are different ways of describing people with respect to their presentations. More importantly, severity is generally related to only one intervention type, while complexity may well indicate multiple, concurrent interventions.

For example, an entrepreneur might have a great idea and the ability to produce and deliver the product that corresponds to the idea but have absolutely no money. This would be a severe shortage of capital or perhaps a severe cash flow problem. Even a very severe need has a relatively simple solution. The solution involves addressing the need, in this case, capital. Thus, a severely undercapitalized business could be saved by an infusion of capital investment. A complex presentation of needs requires a more comprehensive approach. Let's say that another entrepreneur has some capital (although not enough), but also has problems with production and distribution. Now, to get that business going, the intervention has to be multifaceted. A simple influx of capital investment is insufficient.

Applications in health care might similarly distinguish between severity and complexity. A person might have severe diabetes. That person would require intensive treatment. However, a person with less severe diabetes might also have heart disease, be depressed, and have limited social support and unstable housing. This second person, although his or her diabetes is less severe, might well be more difficult to treat because the health circumstance is complex.

Traditional psychometric measurement approaches focus on the careful measurement of severity. The scaling of items on latent continua is an exercise in the measurement of severity when applied to a service need. Although the concept of complexity is seldom explicit in traditional measurement approaches, the manner in which traditional measurement approach this construct handle complexity requires the creation of multiple scaled measure. Thus, the Minnesota Multiphasic Personality Inventory (MMPI, Tellegen et al., 2003) provides a profile of constructs (e.g., eight validity scales and ten clinical scales), each measured with carefully scaled items. The challenge is that the MMPI-A has 478 items (there is a "short" form with only 350 items). The greater the ability to assess complexity, the more different things have to be measured. When multiple items are required to effectively measure each construct, then the response burden increases geometrically.

One of the reasons severity has eclipsed complexity in traditional approaches to measurement is that complexity requires a different statistical approach. Sometimes computation convenience drives applications in science. For example, the Central Limit Theorem was a major break through for statistical analyses as it provided a computational convenience in a time well before computers assisted the calculation of complex statistical analyses. By assuming a normal distribution for sampling distributions given a large enough sample, easier to compute statistical techniques became available. I'm old enough to have had professors when I was in graduate school who spent entire semesters calculating a single regression equation. A factor analysis could take a year to complete. In the absence of computers, linear concepts are appealing from an analytical perspective alone.

Complexity, on the other hand, is not a linear concept. Although one can speak of degrees of complexity, such wording often means different combinations of things, combined in different ways that makes action less clear or more difficult. Since it is not a linear construct, the Central Limit Theorem may not help us in the analysis of complexity. By their design at the individual item level, communimetric tools are intended to allow them to function as indicators of complexity. Currently the most widely used examples of complexity indicators comes from the work with decision support (see Chaps. 3, 5, and 6).

The presentation of the first four chapters of this book has been to provide the reader with an understanding of the background and conceptual framework for communimetrics. While such theoretical discussions are important, often understanding comes from examples. The next three chapters describe three different communimetric tools in an effort to clarify how the concepts described so far are translated into the development and use of measures in various human service enterprises.

Chapter 5
The Child and Adolescent Needs and Strengths

You could describe the Child and Adolescent Needs and Strengths (CANS) as the first communimetric tool. But actually, the experiences taken from the development and implemention of the CANS led to the creation of the communication-based theory of measurement. The journey from a measure of psychiatric case mix used in a planning study in the late 1980s to a practice framework for the child-serving system resulted in collaborations with literally thousands of professionals, parents, and youth who informed the evolution of the approach. The story of the development of the CANS is really the story of the evolution of the communimetric theory of measurement.

A Developmental History

In 1986, prospective payment was the new big thing in health care. At the time, close to one-fourth of the gross national product was being spent on health care and about one-fourth of that was spent on behavioral health care. This expenditure level was described as a health care crisis. Cost containment was considered a viable strategy. Prospective payment, whereby a hospital was paid an episode of care rate based on the characteristics of the patient using diagnostic related groups (DRG), was implemented in Medicare. Diagnostic related groups worked fairly well with medical/surgical patients (e.g., Safran, Porter, Slack, & Bleich, 1987). Cost differences were relatively consistent and predictable between a hip replacement and a hernia repair. Diagnostic related groups did not work for psychiatric hospitalization. Since psychiatry has few, if any, procedures (e.g., electroconvulsive therapy [ECT] remains available, but is rarely used), length of stay is the primary determinant of the cost of a stay in a psychiatric hospital. There was almost no relationship between diagnostic groupings and psychiatric hospital length of stay. Around this time, with colleagues, I published a study predicting psychiatric hospital length of stay and found that the single best predictor was the attending psychiatrist (Lyons, O'Mahoney, & Larson, 1991). In other words, practice pattern variation exceeded any other predictor. The psychiatrist predicted 12% of the variation in length of stay. Shortly after I completed this study, I was talking with Joe Feinglass, a colleague in the Department of Medicine, and he reported the identical size of practice pattern

J.S. Lyons, *Communimetrics: A Communication Theory of Measurement in Human Service Settings*,
DOI 10.1007/978-0-387-92822-7_5, © Springer Science+Business Media, LLC 2009

effect for internal medicine—12%. The big difference was in his work; diagnosis accounted for around 40% of the variation. In my study, DRG only accounted for 4%. That conversation triggered a thought. Maybe applying a health services model in which diagnosis is the primary clinical variable is inappropriate for mental health services research. Perhaps factors other than diagnosis would drive decision making about the use of psychiatric hospitalization and, therefore, predict costs.

But that realization created a new challenge. To do this type of services research you need information on thousands of cases. This research is not like clinical trials or experimental psychopathology studies, which routinely publish studies with samples of less than 100 subjects. In services research you utilize large database to pursue the policy-relevant questions. Because these databases are usually collected for other purposes, such as billing or utilization management, they are called convenience databases in health services research. They are used because they are convenient to use. But convenience databases in behavioral health only had psychiatric diagnoses. Consequently, if we were going to create a large database that contained information relevant to the actual decision making in the field, we would need to create a measurement process that was easy, efficient, and meaningful to the clinician so that it could be available in large databases to match with other heath services information.

When I worked with the Department of Medicine for a year, I was exposed to Susan Horn's work on the severity of illness (Horn, 1983). I was very impressed with how she was able to formalize a measurement strategy that could be applied to medical chart data in a fashion that was reliable and meaningful. I had been trained in graduate school to mistrust any measurement taken from clinical documentation as "too soft for science." When I saw how her system worked I thought that she had cleverly overcome the inherent limitations of her data source by simplifying the structure of her measurement process.

I met with a number of psychiatrists and crisis workers individually and reviewed the existing literature on psychiatric emergency services and psychiatric hospitalization. I also reviewed the standards for involuntary admission into the hospital since, at the time, these criteria (i.e., danger to self, danger to others, inability to care for oneself) were becoming the new standard for medical necessity. During this process, I came across an unpublished measure called the Whittington Index, which I liked for its simplicity and focus on matters relevant to psychiatric crisis services. From these experiences I crafted a measure I called the Severity of Psychiatric Illness (SPI), since the framework and even the four-point scales were borrowed from Susan Horn's approach. My experience of the four-point scales is that they did not demand more precision than what was often available in the medical charts. My thinking was that if it was in the chart, the person noting it thought it was important. So if the SPI could simply quantify the information routinely available in the medical chart, it would have the potential to be easily adopted in prospective use. The capacity for widespread prospective use was critical to any success in getting better mental health indicators in large billing databases to support mental health services research.

The SPI was quite accurate in terms of predicting decisions to admit patients into the psychiatric hospital and also predicted hospital outcomes. It was reasonably accurate for predicting hospital length of stay (Lyons, Colletta, Devens, & Finkel, 1995; Lyons, Kisiel, Dulcan, Cohen, & Chesler 1997). It has been translated into Spanish, Dutch, and German, and published in these languages as well. The success of the SPI in modeling the clinical rationale of psychiatric crisis services set the stage for the development of the CANS by establishing credibility to the basic measurement approach.

In 1995, the Illinois Department of Children and Family Services (IDCFS) had a major challenge. They had 55,000 children in care and a budget of about $1.5 billion. About one-third of these dollars was tied up in behavioral health care. For a managed behavioral health firm that would be a very appealing financial situation. Further, about 80% of the $450 million invested in behavioral health was spent on psychiatric hospitalizations and residential treatment, leaving only a relatively small amount for community-based services. This disparity led to the evolution of a two-tiered system, whereby children and youth would not be served in their communities and then would end up hospitalized because community services weren't available. The very fact that they were hospitalized became an indicator that they needed a "higher level of care," i.e., residential treatment. Thus, after a couple of hospitalizations with little community follow-up, these children and youth were often referred to residential treatment. Further complicating the problem was the fact that providers were generally located where people wanted to go to work, but children with child welfare involvement generally live in the poorest communities in the state (Lyons, Mintzer, Kisiel, & Shallcross, 1998).

A new director, Jess McDonald, was named to head IDCFS, and he wanted to address this problem. An important aspect of the solution would be to create more services in the communities where the children lived. Service creation, however, requires the investment of new dollars. It would have been great if the legislature was ready to give IDCFS more money to develop these intensive community-based services, but at the time of his appointment, Mr. McDonald could not even get confirmed by the Illinois state senate. The *Chicago Tribune* was running a series called "Death of Our Children," which inventoried a series of missteps by IDCFS workers. So under the circumstances, the legislature did not want to "put good money after bad," and decided to force the new director to make changes without any additional resources. They only agreed to allow him to reinvest anything he was able to save. This promise proved to be enough.

The Illinois Department of Children and Family Services leadership decided that their only viable approach was to use a community reinvestment strategy in which they moved children and youth from expensive residential treatment programs ($100–$600/day) into community placements, such as foster homes and return to families. Further, they would bring children and youth from out of state placement to replace those moved into the community from in-state providers to lessen the financial impact of the reduce residential placements on in-state providers. In undertaking this project, they explained their strategy to residential providers and then asked the providers to nominate children and youth to participate in this process of return to the community. This strategy proved to be a costly misstep. Unfortunately, since without checks and balances, all institutions function at the convenience of the institution, residential providers sometimes failed to nominate children and youth who were doing well (e.g., "We are helping. Don't disrupt their treatment."); instead, nominated children and youth who still required intensive services (e.g., "We are not helping. Maybe you can help."). Thus, the provider nomination process sometimes resulted in the identification of exactly the wrong children and youth for return to the community.

An absolutely tragic event happened in which a very high-need youth who was in a very intensive out of state placement was identified for return (i.e., they weren't able to help him). Unfortunately, he had grandparents who loved him. They said that if no one else was willing, they would try. They lived in a small town, and 6 weeks after they moved this young man from a very intensive residential program to living with his grandparents, he murdered both of them. This story is a tragic example of how not to manage a service system. This young man needed an intensive service setting. He needed to be in a safe, structured, residential treatment center. But, because a community placement was available and there was pressure to reduce the number of youth in placements, the decision was made to step this young man down to live with relatives.

Given my experience in using structured assessments to model the clinical rationale of the psychiatric crisis services, I was invited to participate in the design of a process for identifying which children and youth could return to the community without tragedy. Since I was unfamiliar with the child welfare system, and relatively unfamiliar with children's behavioral health, we initiated the project by holding a number of focus groups in which the discussion was focused on identifying exactly what characteristics of children and youth should inform good decision making in the child welfare system.

In these discussions, a three-dimensional model emerged. Symptoms of behavioral and emotional disorders tended to inform choice of treatment approach. If a child was hallucinating, one should consider psychotropic medication. If a child was depressed or anxious even the Surgeon General Report (2001) recommended a psychotherapeutic approach (i.e., talking). But if a child is oppositional, every evidence-based practice suggests an environment intervention focus on the caregivers (Brestan & Eyberg, 1998; Kazdin, 2005). But knowledge of symptoms does not fully inform the intensity with which services should be applied. In fact, high-risk behaviors become an important consideration to how intensively an intervention is needed. Factors such as suicide, violence, or sexual aggression influence intensity of service/level of care decisions. However, symptoms and risks do not fully inform decision making in the child-serving system. Knowing that a child is depressed and suicidal, you might still feel comfortable serving him or her in a community setting, but only if the parent or caregiver was knowledgeable and able to provide appropriate supervision, etc.

The result of these focus group discussions was the creation of a tool that included the identified three dimensions described in the preceding—symptoms, risks, and caregiver capacity. The original version was called the Childhood Severity of Psychiatric Illness (CSPI). Table 5.1 contains the items included in the original CSPI. Based on the SPI in structure, the items of the CSPI were designed

Table 5.1 Items included on the Original Childhood Severity of Psychiatric Illness

Symptoms
Neuropsychiatric disturbance
Emotional disturbance
Conduct disturbance
Oppositional behavior
Impulsivity
Contextual consistency of symptoms
Temporal consistency of symptoms
Risk factors
Suicide risk
Danger to others
Elopement risk
Crime/delinquency
Sexual aggression
Functioning
School dysfunction
Family dysfunction
Peer dysfunction
Comorbidity
Adjustment to original trauma/separation
Medical
Substance abuse
Severity of abuse
Sexual development
Learning and developmental disabilities
Systems factors
Caregiver ability to provide supervision
Caregiver motivation for change
Caregiver knowledge of child
Placement safety
Community capacity for WRAP services
Multisystem needs

to assess the unique clinical characteristics of children and adolescents in care. The basic design of the SPI worked for this project because it was essential to first answer the primary question, "Are there children and youth currently placed in residential treatment who do not need to be there?" Susan Horn and her colleagues had already demonstrated that it was possible to obtain information relevant to decision making from chart review provided the tool was designed appropriately. By using the structure of the SPI, we could use the CSPI to review the records of children and youth currently in residential treatment to rapidly assess the potential appropriateness of these placements.

We then applied the CSPI to a stratified random sample of children and youth in residential treatment in Illinois (Lyons, Mintzer, Kisiel, & Shallcross, 1998). In this review, we found that 13% of children and youth had never engaged in any of the five high-risk behaviors. About 20% had a history of engaging in at least one of these high-risk behaviors, but not in the time period immediately prior to the most recent admission into residential treatment. So, fully one-third of children and youth in residential placement reasonably could be stepped down into the community without intensive services already in place.

Once the findings of this study were accepted, IDCFS designed a process to reduce the number of children and youth based on their CSPI profiles. A one-third reduction was accomplished within 18 months by simultaneously applying a simple decision model for both placement into residential treatment and step down from residential treatment back to a community placement. Basically, the original CSPI decision model for residential treatment was that one needed at least one 2 or 3 on at least one Symptom need *and* at least one 2 or 3 on at least one risk behavior. It should be noted that this simple model represents an *extremely* low threshold to residential placement that no jurisdiction uses anymore. It was a starting point to initiate a system transformation. A shifting decision model is an example of planned incrementalism. A staged approach to system change can be an effective and sustainable change strategy and an essential premise of this approach is to not get too far ahead of the field. Reducing the number of children and youth in residential treatment by one-third was seen as sufficient to fund the development of intensive community services in the state. This change was difficult enough for residential providers in the state; a more dramatic reduction would have been far more difficult to achieve.

The community reinvestment strategy envisioned by DCFS leadership became a reality over the next 2 years, with the number of children and youth placed in expensive residential treatment centers dropping from a peak of more than 6,000 in 1995 to about 4,000 18 months later. At the writing of this book, approximately 1,600 children and youth are currently in residential placements through the Illinois DCFS.

The reduction of more than 2,000 admissions to residential treatment had major consequences to the child-serving system beyond freeing up resources to fund intensive community services. Since the average residential treatment center has about 50 beds, the success of this initiative resulted in the inevitable closure of a number of programs. As anyone who has ever worked in the public sector will tell you, this type of dramatic change process can be fairly easy to derail. All that would have had to happen is for a few chief executive officers of large residential programs to call their legislators and complain that the state is forcing the closure of a business(es) in the legislator's district. Politicians use their influence to bring business in their districts. State-funded child welfare business is as good as any other, particularly in rural areas that have been hurt by shifts in agriculture and the closing of manufacturing plants. Children don't vote, but employees of residential treatment centers do. Thus, political contingencies often favor human service providers over state bureaucrats. Despite the ease with which this complaint can be used effectively, it did not happen in this process to any great extent. In fact, a number of facilities closed voluntarily and, where possible, began to shift their business model towards developing intensive community service programs.

I have been convinced that a primary driving factor in the long-term success of the community reinvestment strategy was that the process was always about what was in the best interests of children. This focus on a shared vision of the child-serving system and our ability to keep the children and youths' needs at the forefront of the planning and change process through the development and use of the CSPI was a fundamental reason for the success of the initiative. This experience is captured by the constitutive concept of communication—creating a shared meaning about how to best serve children and then representing it in a measurement process to guide the implementation and reinforce the shared meaning.

Following this experience, Northwestern University decided to exercise intellectual property rights over the CSPI and entered a contract with the Psychological Corporation. This arrangement was not really satisfactory for any of the parties as the company sought the CSPI to sell a managed care/outcomes management software system that never really took off. The university only made a few hundred dollars, half of which they generously shared with the Mental Health Services and Policy Program. The Psychological Corporation has since released the copyright on the CSPI and related tools.

Despite the commercial failure of the CSPI, saving millions of dollars for reinvestment in community services without the use of a managed care company, garner a lot of attention in the child-serving system. Because of the success of the Illinois initiative to reduce residential treatment utilization, I began to get invited to national meetings. In the process of being included by the national leadership at that time in the child-serving system, I became exposed to issues that had not come up in the Illinois project. Primary among these issues was strengths and strength-based planning. During the Illinois focus groups and discussions, the issue of strengths was never raised. However, in the late 1990s, strengths had become a very hot topic on the U.S. national child-serving scene.

The concept of strengths is that children, youth, and families have assets that can help them through challenging times. Focusing on identifying, developing, and using these assets is the heart of strength-based planning. Intensive community treatment approaches, called wraparound services, embraced strength-based planning a guiding premise to its approach to working with families (c.f., VanDenBerg & Grealish, 1998).

At that time there was considerable tension between advocates of strength-based approaches and what were considered traditional clinical approaches that diagnosed psychopathology and worked to directly treat the identified symptoms of psychiatric disorders. Strength-based advocates called this deficit based, and decried that it was out of date and out of touch with the needs of children and families. Clinical advocates considered the strength-based advocates to be Pollyanna and frankly naïve.

Given the strong interest in strengths at the national level, my colleagues and I created a brief strengths assessment to be used in parallel to the CSPI. We called the measure the Child and Adolescent Strengths Assessment (CASA; Lyons, Uziel-Miller, Reyes, & Sokol, 2000). We used it in a project in Florida investigating a bundled-rated payment methodology in Medicaid to pilot this measure. In studying the relationship between the CASA and the CSPI we discovered that strengths and symptoms both have significant relationships to level of functioning and the likelihood of high-risk behavior, but these relationships are completely independent of one another. In other words, the more symptomatic a child, the lower his or her level of functioning and the more likely he or she will engage in high-risk behavior. Completely independent of symptoms levels, the more strength a child has, the higher his or her level of functioning and the less likely he or she is to engage in high-risk behavior. Hence, both the clinical and the strength-based advocates were right in their perspectives, but wrong in their disrespect for the others' viewpoint. The clear implication of these findings is the optimally effective treatment of children and youth should include both efforts to reduce symptomatology *and* efforts to use and build strengths. Based on the results of this study, the CANS was created in an effort to integrate the clinical and strengths perspective into a single assessment approach.

The very first state-wide implementation of the CANS started in Florida within 1 year of this project; however, it was with the next project that the shift of the CANS to a communimetric measurement tool actually occurred. I was invited to work with Allegheny County, PA (e.g., Pittsburgh) on tailoring the CANS for their project, which was a funded through the Substance Abuse and Mental Health Service Administration (SAMHSA) as a system of care site. Substance Abuse and Mental Health Service Administration funds many jurisdictions around the country to develop intensive community-based services using system of care philosophy (Stroul & Freidman, 1986). Allegheny County wanted to use the CANS as an integrated assessment process within their project.

It is useful to consider the nature of system of care projects as it relates to the evolution of the CANS. System of care philosophy is articulated in the guiding principles and core values listed in Table 5.2. One of the implications of this philosophy is that parents and youth should be involved in all aspects of the service system.

Table 5.2 Core Values and Guiding Principles of the Child and Adolescent Support Services Programs (CASSP)

CASSP core values

1. The system of care should be child centered, with the needs of the child and family dictating the types and mix of services provided.
2. The system of care should be community-based, with the locus of services as well as management and decision-making responsibility resting at the community level.

CASSP guiding principles

1. Emotionally disturbed children should have access to a comprehensive array of services that address the child's physical, emotional, social, and educational needs.
2. Emotionally disturbed children should receive individualized services in accordance with the unique needs and potentials of each child, and guided by an individualized service plan.
3. Emotionally disturbed children should receive services within the least restrictive, most normative environment that is clinically appropriate.
4. The families and surrogate families of emotionally disturbed children should be full participants in all aspects of the planning and delivery of services.
5. Emotionally disturbed children should receive services that are integrated, with linkages between child-caring agencies and programs and mechanisms for planning, developing, and coordinating services.
6. Emotionally disturbed children should be provided with case management or similar mechanisms to ensure that multiple services are delivered in a coordinated and therapeutic manner, and that they can move through the system of services in accordance with their changing needs.

(continued)

Table 5.2 (continued)

7. Early identification and intervention for children with emotional problems should be promoted by the system of care in order to enhance the likelihood of positive outcomes.
8. Emotionally disturbed children should be ensured smooth transitions to the adult services system as they reach maturity.
9. The rights of emotionally disturbed children should be protected; and effective advocacy efforts for emotionally disturbed children and youth should be promoted.
10. Emotionally disturbed children should receive services without regard to race, religion, national origin, sex, physical disability, or other characteristics, and services should be sensitive and responsive to cultural differences and special needs.

Source: Adapted from the Child and Adolescent Support Services Programs guidelines (Stroul, 1993).

Allegheny County had very strong family representation through a group of parent advocates led by Julie Hdalio. The project director, Gwen White, wanted the family members to be the driving force behind the tailoring of the CANS. So, I and the project evaluator, Mary Beth Rauktis, met with the family members multiple times to hammer out relevant items and language that they felt captured the needs and strengths of their children in a way that reduced stigma and judgment coming from professionals. The constitutive communication process initiated with the creation of the CSPI was taken to an entirely different level by this process. The explicit effort was to develop a measure that could serve as a mechanism for creating shared meaning for families and service professionals in the service delivery process. We referred to it as developing a common language.

As importantly, walking back from lunch during one of these marathon meetings, I was casually talking to the lead parent, Julie Hdalio. To establish the context, the levels of the CSPI was defined using more traditional Likert-type rating scales of None, Mild, Moderate, and Severe. But in training first in the CSPI and then with the CANS, I had often mentioned that you could also think about things from a service planning perspective of No Evidence, Watchful Waiting/Prevention, Action, and Immediate/Intensive Action. These ratings were not explicit aspects of the CANS at that time, just alternative ways of understanding the Likert ratings. During this conversation, Julie told me emphatically that the things she really liked about the CANS were, in fact, the action levels I had described in my presentation. She said that the action levels would make immediate sense to parents. Parents experience many assessments of their children and often do not know how to translate these assessments into what should happen next. Parents then struggle to hold providers accountable for following up on the findings of the assessment. She felt that the action levels made the relation between assessment and services planning and receipt transparent, and that was the primary value of the approach.

By that time the CANS had evolved into a tool that could be tailored to different circumstances, including both needs and strengths in an effort to integrate competing conceptualization, and now was action-oriented in its item structure. So the Allegheny County version of the CANS was the first full communimetric measure evolved to be the shared meaning in the child-serving system between parents and professionals and facilitate communication within the service planning process.

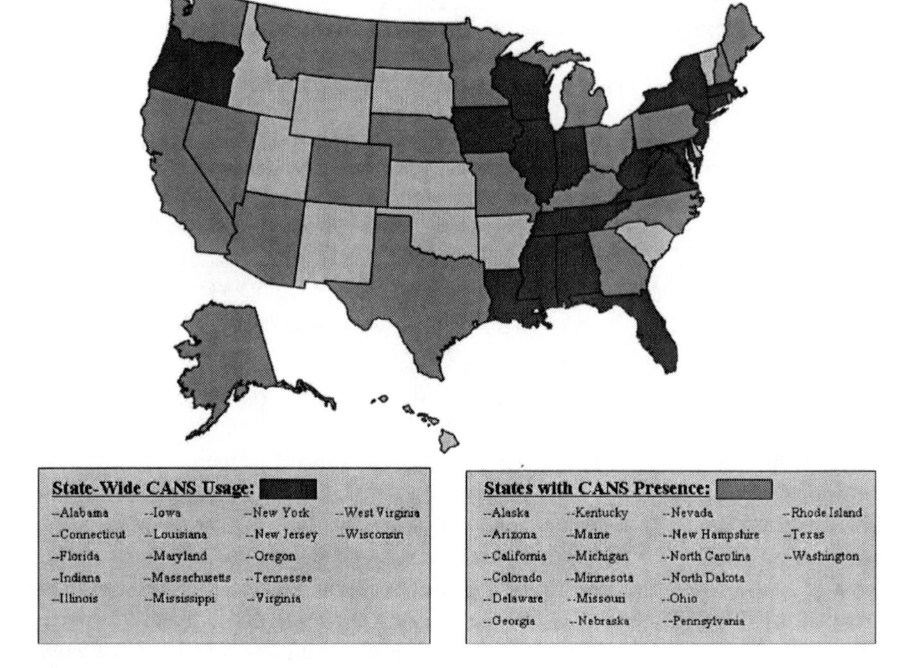

Figure 5.1 CANS usage in the United States

The number of jurisdictions and agencies implementing of the CANS has continued to increase since that time. Figure 5.1 displays all of the current North American applications by jurisdiction at the time of this writing. Additional states are considering state-wide implementations. Learning collaborative to support training and analysis and interpretation have been initiative to support the mass collaboration model of dissemination of innovation (see Chap. 8).

Measurement Characteristics of the Child and Adolescent Needs and Strengths

Reliability

There is substantial research and implementations establishing the reliability of the CANS. Anderson et al. (2003) demonstrated that the CANS is reliable at the item level both prospectively and using field audit methods. In a variety of published research, the reliability of the CANS as a case review method has been reported to be about 0.85 (Lyons, 2004). Reliability testing prospectively (with two ratings describing the same child) has been observed to around 0.90 (Lyons, 2004).

Use of the CANS generally requires formal certification which means that trainees must complete a test case vignette with reliability (intraclass correlation) of 0.70 or above. There are more than 30,000 individuals around the world who have been certified in the reliability use of the CANS. Following a standard half-day training, 80% to 90% achieve this level of reliability on their first attempt. The majority of those who fail initially, achieve reliability on their second test vignette.

At this point, there is no doubt that the CANS can be a reliable measure. However, it also is true that it can be used unreliably. In our experience the essential to ongoing reliability are the factors discussed early in this text—use, transparency, and ongoing monitoring.

Validity

Several types of validity have been studied and established for the CANS. Face validity is demonstrated by its widespread acceptance in a large variety of child-serving systems. There has been remarkably little resistance from family advocates and clinicians for most implementations. The approach clearly makes sense to those working directly with children and families. Most resistance to CANS implementations actually comes from individuals schooled in traditional psychometric measurement approaches who are uncomfortable with the communimetric approach.

In terms of construct validity, CANS dimension scores have been shown to correlate with other measures of child status, such as the CAFAS and the Child Behavior Checklist (Lyons, 2004). These correlations are highest when the context is the same for all children in the sample. When some children are in a residential placement and others are in the community, the correlation between the CANS and the CAFAS is much lower, as the CANS does not report setting effects as meeting the needs of children, whereas the CAFAS does (Lyons, 2004). In other words, a child who is going to school at a campus-based residential program because staff wake him or her up and ensure that he or she attends the on-campus school would be seen as fine on the CAFAS, but on the CANS could still be seen as having school attendance needs.

Utility validity has been reported. The CANS has been widely embedded in treatment and service planning processes and is widely used in supervision and quality improvement (O'Brien & Schneider, 2007). There have been many reports of improved attention to strengths resulting in the use of this structured assessment process (e.g., Craig & MacIntyre, 2008). Rawal, Anderson, Romansky, and Lyons (2008) have demonstrated that this approach can reduce and practically eliminate racial disparities in psychiatric hospital admissions.

Research documenting the decision validity is growing; some is be reported in the following. There is a growing body of research that has not yet been published that documents that CANS-recommended program placements result in improved outcomes (Hancock, 2008). Lyons, Woltman, Martinovich & Hancock, 2009 reported that using the CANS decision model to assist in placements in residential treatment resulted in improved within-episode outcomes for residential treatment providers.

Scoring Options

There are three strategies for scoring the CANS. The first is the simplest. Since the CANS is designed to be reliable at the item level and research has documented this level of reliability, it is completely legitimate to analyze information from individual items. Individual item analyses are useful both for describing the characteristics of children, youth, and families presenting to a program or the system or for monitoring outcomes from episodes of care. Reporting the percent of children or youth who move from an actionable level of need (2 or 3) to a 0 or 1 is one widely used strategy for reporting met need.

The second scoring strategy is by CANS dimensions. The recommended scoring strategy is to average available items and multiply by 10. This creates 30-point scales in which a 0 is a child or youth with all 0 ratings on the items within a dimension and a 30 would be a child or youth with all 3 ratings on the items within a dimension. Dimension scores are quite useful for program evaluation applications to allow for the study of the effects of different interventions (Lyons, Griffin, Jenuwine, Shasha, & Quintenz, 2003; Weiner, Schneider, & Lyons, 2008).

The third strategy is to create a single score to represent the functional status of a child or youth. This approach is not recommended, but is possible if one only utilizes a subset of the items. Specifically, it is possible to create a single score by combining items from behavioral/emotional needs, risk behaviors, and functioning. These items form a reasonable scale in traditional psychometric terms. It is not a good idea to include strengths or caregiver items in this total scale, and these two dimensions represent very different constructs than the three child/youth specific need dimensions. Doucette's (2007) scaling of the comprehensive version of the CANS supports this scoring option.

Psychometric Scale Properties

Once you choose to score the CANS by adding items within dimension you must subject it to the same measurement standards as any psychometric measure. Interestingly, it appears that when you do analyze the CANS from traditional psychometric perspectives, you find that you can, in fact, score it by dimensions and use these indices just like you would a traditional measure designed from a psychometric perspective.

For example, Table 5.3 presents a correlation matrix for behavioral health items from the comprehensive version of the CANS. In addition, the item to total correlation between each item and the total behavioral health score (item average × 10) is provided. Review of these data suggests that all items fit the standard classical test theory of at least an item-total correlation coefficient of 0.30. The highest correlations are the disruptive behavior items that are the most common behavioral health needs, but these correlations do not top 0.70. Cronbach's alpha for this set of items is 0.70 on this

Table 5.3 Item Analysis of the Behavioral/Emotional Needs of the CANS Comprehensive Based on 6,010 Initial Assessments in New Jersey

Item	Total	Psychosis	Anxiety	Depression	AdjTrauma	Impulse	Oppositional	Conduct	Anger
Psychosis	0.34								
Anxiety	0.55	0.23							
Depression	0.54	0.21	0.46						
AdjTrauma	0.44	0.14	0.29	0.31					
Impulse	0.64	0.14	0.24	0.14	0.11				
Oppositional	0.58	0.03	0.14	0.15	0.06	0.47			
Conduct	0.64	0.08	0.13	0.12	0.07	0.39	0.54		
Anger	0.67	0.08	0.18	0.14	0.11	0.44	0.61	0.43	
Substance	0.30	–0.03	0.01	0.10	–0.06	0.03	0.15	0.22	0.08

sample of 6,010 children and youth. Under classical test theory, there characteristics are sufficient to justify using a total behavioral/emotional needs score. Substance use has some inter-item correlations that might lead one to suggest it not be included in the total score; however, its item-total correlation is sufficient. It is probably the relationship of this need item to the age of the youth that dimensions its correlation with some other needs.

Table 5.4 presents a similar correlation matrix for the strength items. The Cronbach's alpha for these items was 0.71, again sufficient to justify using a scale score. Inter-item correlations are all consistent with a sound classically designed measure.

Based on these analyses, a classically trained psychometrician might argue for the shortening of the behavioral/emotional needs scale to just the three highly correlated disruptive behavior items (i.e., oppositional, conduct, and anger control) or to specifically exclude substance use (i.e., It has a zero or even low negative correlation with some other items.). A communimetric approach would never support such a strategy. The inclusion of items has to do with the work that must be done, not the statistical relationship among items. The measure does not exist only to generate a total score. The measure exists to support the work with the human service enterprise. Although disruptive behavior is more common, some children and youth have major mental illness or depression and/or anxiety, and different treatment approaches are indicated for these different needs. Good treatment planning requires the inclusion of all of these items separately; therefore, changing the measure because of the statistics would be misguided. This is a fundamental difference between a communimetric tool and a psychometric tool. You do not use inter-item performance indicators to guide measurement development—only to guide scoring options.

Rasch Modeling the Child and Adolescent Needs and Strengths

Item response theory and Rasch modeling specifically is another strategy for understanding the scale properties of a communimetric tool when you wish to aggregate it into scores. This section presents a Rasch scaling of the Illinois IDCFS version of the CANS. This version can be found in Appendix A. A sample of 4,182 children and youth at entry into the IDCFS system were used for these analyses. It should be noted that at entry into IDCFS it is anticipated that children and youth have lower needs than if one were to sample other points in the system. For example, children and youth who disrupt from regular foster care have higher needs (Chor, 2008). Children and youth who stay in the custody of the state longer have higher needs than those who return to permanency rapidly. These sample variations in the frequency of needs has an impact on how items scale. Given the design of the CANS, a sample of children and youth at entry into state custody would be expected to populate the lower end of the full distribution of children and youth who might be assessed with the CANS.

For the sample at entry into the IDCFS system, when all items are scaled together this version of the CANS was an item separation of 2.69, which translates

Table 5.4 Item Analysis of Strength Items from the CANS-Comprehensive Based on 6,010 Initial Assessments in New Jersey

Item	Total	Family	Education	Community	Interpersonal	Optimism	Permanence	Spiritual	Talents
Family	0.52								
Education	0.45	0.12							
Community	0.64	0.22	0.20						
Interpersonal	0.51	0.29	0.20	0.32					
Optimism	0.58	0.27	0.20	0.29	0.40				
Permanence	0.47	0.31	0.08	0.24	0.18	0.18			
Spiritual	0.57	0.16	0.13	0.37	0.17	0.22	0.15		
Talents	0.61	0.21	0.21	0.32	0.32	0.29	0.14	0.27	
Vocational	0.50	0.09	0.13	0.20	0.24	0.16	0.09	0.14	0.31

into a Cronbach's alpha of about 0.88, which is adequate from a scaling perspective. Thus, the overall CANS is scalable using this model. From a Rasch perspective, the most "noise" was generated by the 1 level rating (i.e., watchful waiting/prevention for the need items). This finding may relate to the multiple ways this level is used (e.g., suspicion, need for assessment, and history).

The success of Rasch scaling, like other psychometric approaches, is somewhat dependent on the length of the scale. More items tend to scale better than fewer items. However, it is important to scale needs and strengths separately, as they use a different set of action levels. Further, caregiver items are assessing a very different construct than those designed for describing children and youth. Therefore, separate analyses were accomplished for each domain of the CANS.

For the Strengths dimension the item separation statistic was a 1.81, which translates into a Child Reliability of 0.77. This is certainly adequate. Table 5.5 presents the item fit statistics for this scale. Review of this table demonstrates that Vocational Strengths is the only item with a fit statistic outside the recommended range. This finding should not be surprising because Vocational Strengths are not applicable for children and young adolescents, but quite relevant for older youth. It may be advisable not to include Vocational Strengths in Strength dimension scores if children and young adolescents are predominant in the sample. Figure 5.2 present the probability distribution across the four levels of each item within the Strengths dimension. Again, the structure is adequate with the 1 rating providing the most noise.

Table 5.6 provides an item analysis for a combination of behavioral/emotional, risk behaviors, and life domain functioning items. Together these items hang together reasonably well as an overall measure of a child/youth's functional status with a separation index of 1.98 and a reliability of 0.80; however, review of the individual items reveals three items: Job Functioning, Medical Functioning, and Developmental as not fitting particularly well. This finding should not be surprising as only a small subset of youth are working, severe medical problems are rare at entry into child welfare, and the developmental item is a static indicator of mental retardation or developmental delay. The interpretation of these finding from a scaling perspective is that you would not includes these three items in a total score to be used in an outcome analysis, but that a single scale combining these items to give an overall functional status measure for children and youth would be feasible.

It is important to remember that these analyses were done using the population of children and youth at their entry into child welfare. There are many children and youth with minimal needs at this particular time. Since psychometric techniques require variation in order to achieve good statistical performance of the items, this sample is not optimal for these scaling approaches. When a broader sample of children and youth actually in service are used for scaling purposes, the performance of the CANS dimensions improves dramatically. In a scaling of 6,010 children and youth from New Jersey, Doucette (2007) found that the comprehensive version of the CANS had good scaling properties for each of the dimensions and that a combination of behavioral/emotional, risk behaviors, and functioning made a well functioning total score. Strengths did not scale with the other items, which should

Table 5.5 Rasch Item Fit for the Strengths Domain

					Infit		Outfit		PTMEA	Exact match		
Entry number	Raw score	Count	Measure	Real S.E.	MNSQ	ZSTD	MNSQ	ZSTD	CORR.	OBS (%)	EXP (%)	Strength
22	1,757	4,016	1.0	0.0	1.65	9.9	1.15	3.1	0.53	67.2	68.3	cs_vocational
24	2,644	4,016	0.4	0.0	0.63	−9.9	0.55	−9.9	0.71	71.4	59.0	cs_optimism
25	2,891	4,016	0.3	0.0	0.90	−4.3	0.75	−8.4	0.69	65.7	58.3	cs_talents_interests
21	3,040	4,016	0.2	0.0	1.20	8.0	1.13	3.8	0.62	59.8	56.4	cs_educational
20	3,117	4,016	0.2	0.0	0.80	−9.0	0.84	−5.5	0.67	61.9	56.1	cs_interpersonal
26	3,436	4,016	0.0	0.0	1.24	9.9	1.10	3.3	0.65	55.6	53.7	cs_spiritual_religious
23	3,691	4,016	−0.1	0.0	0.59	−9.9	0.59	−9.9	0.75	65.7	53.3	cs_wellbeing
27	3,883	4,016	−0.2	0.0	0.89	−5.0	0.78	−8.5	0.73	54.7	51.2	cs_community_life
28	5,524	4,016	−0.9	0.0	1.34	9.9	1.46	9.9	0.55	43.8	47.4	cs_relationship_permanence
19	5,882	4,016	−1.0	0.0	1.29	9.9	1.50	9.9	0.55	42.7	47.8	cs_family
MEAN	3,586.5	4,016.0	0.0	0.0	1.05	1.0	0.98	−1.2		58.9	55.1	
S.D	1,199.3	.0	0.6	0.0	0.32	8.8	0.32	7.7		9.2	5.8	

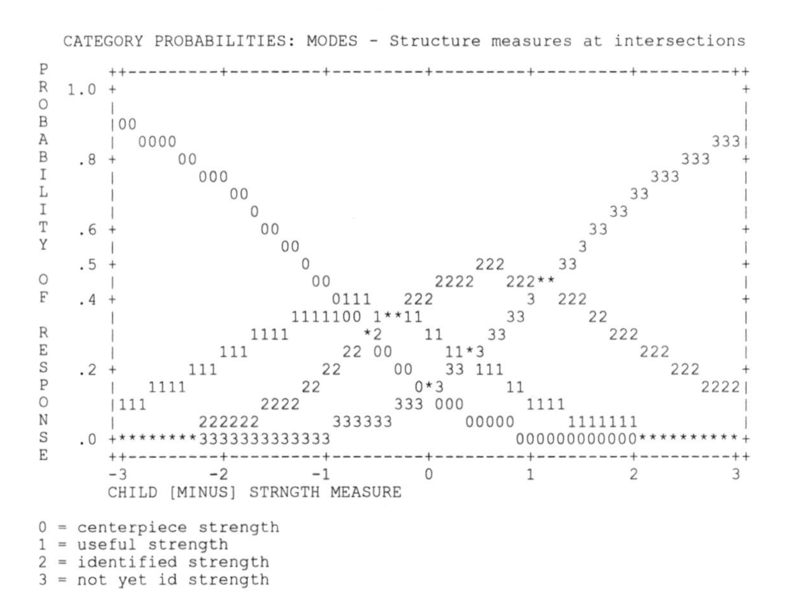

Figure 5.2 Probability structure of the strengths dimension on the Illinois DCFS version of the CANS

be expected given the difference in the definitions of action levels between needs and strengths.

Decision Support for Level of Care and Intensity of Services

As discussed in previous chapters, a well-designed communimetric measure should be able to perform varied tasks within a complex system. The Total Clinical Outcomes Management framework in child and youth services requires the ability of the measure to function as a decision support tool at the program level (Lyons, 2004). This application is generally called level of care or intensity of service decision support. There are a wide variety of these types of decision support model, sometimes referred to as algorithms.

Chap. 4 discussed the difference between the concepts of severity and complexity. It is in the application of a communimetric measure to program level decision support where this distinction is most important. Most other decision support approaches use a severity indictor with a cutoff. For example, with the CAFAS (Hodges & Wotring, 2000) a total score is calculated and different levels of care are recommended for children and youth scoring 120 or above and 80 to 119. The challenge with the severity approach is that it does not necessarily reflect the decision inputs that actually go into good decision making about program eligibility. In fact, most program eligibility models actually reflect complexity rather than severity as primary inputs into decision-making.

Table 5.6 Rasch Scaling Of The Behavioral/Emotional, Risk Behaviors and Functioning Items of the CANS for the Illinois Department of Children and Family Services

					Infit		Outfit		PTMEA	Exact match		
Entry number	Raw score	Count	Measure	Real S.E.	MNSQ	ZSTD	MNSQ	ZSTD	CORR.	OBS (%)	EXP (%)	Strength
67	181	3,793	1.9	0.1	1.04	0.7	0.66	−2.6	0.28	95.5	95.3	Fire setting
63	227	3,793	1.7	0.1	1.11	1.8	0.46	−5.2	0.33	94.9	94.2	Sexual aggression
60	285	3,793	1.4	0.1	0.94	−1.1	0.68	−3.1	0.35	93.0	92.7	Self-mutilation
61	374	3,793	1.1	0.1	0.95	−1.0	0.66	−3.9	0.40	91.5	90.6	Other—self-harm
69	449	3,793	0.8	0.1	1.03	0.7	0.69	−3.9	0.40	89.7	88.9	Sexually reactive behavior
59	454	3,793	0.8	0.1	0.89	−2.8	0.59	−5.4	0.43	89.6	88.8	Suicide risk
18	576	3,793	0.8	0.0	1.09	2.0	0.88	−1.4	0.40	87.2	86.8	Dissociation
65	521	3,793	0.7	0.0	0.89	−2.9	0.47	−8.4	0.47	88.7	87.3	Delinquency
38	533	3,793	0.6	0.0	1.01	0.2	0.66	−5.0	0.44	88.2	87.0	Sexuality
64	547	3,793	0.6	0.0	1.00	0.0	0.63	−5.5	0.46	88.7	86.7	Runaway
37	598	3,793	0.5	0.1	1.36	8.8	1.66	7.6	0.25	82.5	85.7	Physical
35	607	3,793	0.4	0.0	1.07	1.9	0.65	−5.6	0.45	86.9	85.5	Legal
62	689	3,793	0.3	0.0	0.78	−6.9	0.56	−8.1	0.52	87.1	83.9	Danger to others
34	706	3,793	0.2	0.1	1.86	9.9	1.39	5.4	0.36	84.6	83.5	Job functioning
17	1,089	3,793	0.1	0.0	1.23	6.3	0.96	−.6	0.48	77.6	77.9	Numbing
68	925	3,793	−0.1	0.0	0.83	−6.1	0.57	−9.6	0.56	83.8	79.7	Social behavior
41	970	3,793	−0.2	0.0	1.10	3.5	0.90	−2.0	0.49	80.0	78.9	School attendance
16	1,371	3,793	−0.2	0.0	1.22	6.8	1.01	0.2	0.51	72.4	73.4	Avoidance
15	1,390	3,793	−0.2	0.0	1.36	9.9	1.17	3.0	0.48	69.6	73.2	Re-experiencing
66	1,047	3,793	−0.3	0.0	0.70	−9.9	0.50	−9.9	0.62	85.3	77.8	Judgment
39	1,212	3,793	−0.6	0.0	0.85	−5.8	0.68	−8.4	0.60	79.3	75.3	School behavior
32	1,279	3,793	−0.6	0.0	1.49	9.9	1.70	9.9	0.31	61.4	74.3	Developmental
36	1,313	3,793	−0.7	0.0	1.55	9.9	2.19	9.9	0.23	59.1	74.0	Medical
33	1,409	3,793	−0.8	0.0	0.84	−6.8	0.75	−7.1	0.58	75.5	72.7	Recreational
40	1,441	3,793	−0.8	0.0	0.92	−3.1	0.80	−5.7	0.60	76.7	72.4	School achievement

(continued)

Table 5.6 (continued)

					Infit		Outfit		PTMEA	Exact match		
Entry number	Raw score	Count	Measure	Real S.E.	MNSQ	ZSTD	MNSQ	ZSTD	CORR.	OBS (%)	EXP (%)	Strength
30	1,788	3,793	−1.2	0.0	0.92	−3.6	0.92	−2.6	0.58	69.1	68.3	Living situation
31	2,131	3,793	−1.6	0.0	0.68	−9.9	0.66	−9.9	0.69	74.6	65.8	Social function
14	3,772	3,793	−1.9	0.0	1.09	3.8	1.13	4.6	0.66	52.3	54.3	Adjustment to trauma
29	3,313	3,793	−2.6	0.0	0.89	−5.5	0.94	−3.0	0.65	63.6	59.4	Family function
MEAN	1,075.8	3,793.0	0.0	0.0	1.06	0.4	0.88	−2.6		80.3	79.8	
S.D.	825.5	0.0	1.0	0.0	0.26	5.9	0.40	5.6		11.1	9.9	

CANS and Level of Care Recommendations

Residential treatment

The CANS embraces a complexity model in its decision support applications at the program level. Rather than calculating a total score with cutoffs, the logic of complexity dictates that a variety of actionable needs across different domains would influence a decision toward a higher level of care or more intensive treatment intervention. For example, the very first decision algorithm developed from this model was the one used in the residential treatment reform described in the preceding in which the first communimetric tool (CSPI) was developed. As described, that project sought the description of a child or youth who should be served in a residential treatment center. The very first model suggested that in order to place a child in residential treatment, he or should have, at minimum at least one 2 or 3 rating on a symptom of emotional/behavioral disorders AND at least one 2 or 3 on a risk behavior from among the five risk original behaviors as presented in Table 5.1.

Work on decision models has continued and now sophisticated models exist in a number of jurisdictions. The most recent example of the level of care model used in child welfare in Illinois is contained in Table 5.7.

A growing body of validity information demonstrates that the decision models result in better outcomes than decisions that are not consistent with the CANS recommended level of care. For example, in a sample of 1,020 children placed through a child/family team model in child welfare in Illinois (Child and Youth Investment Team, CAYIT), the CANS is used to advise the team, but the team is free to choose any placement. So some children are placed at levels of care lower

Table 5.7 CANS Comprehensive Decision Support Model for the Illinois Department of Children and Family Services

Option 1. Services in Foster care (SFC)
Criterion 1.1: Child is 5 or younger and receives a 2 on at least one of the following:
Communication
Failure to thrive
Regulatory problems
Pica
Substance exposure
Criterion 1.2: At least one 2 or 3 on any of the behavioral/emotional needs items:
Psychosis
Attention deficit/impulse
Depression
Anxiety
Oppositional behavior
Antisocial behavior
Attachment
Adjustment to trauma
Substance use

(continued)

Table 5.7 (continued)

Anger control
Affect dysregulation
Eating disturbance
Behavioral regression
Somatization
To be suggested for SFC referral, a child must either meet Criteria 1.1 OR 1.2
Option 2. Specialized Foster Care
Criterion 2.1: A rating of 2 or 3 on medical/physical or somatization
Criterion 2.2: At least one 2 or 3 on one of the following
Psychosis
Attention deficit/impulse
Depression
Anxiety
Oppositional behavior
Antisocial behavior
Anger control
Attachment
Adjustment to trauma
Substance use
Affect dysregulation
Eating disturbance
Behavioral regression
Criterion 2.3: A rating of 3 on at least one of the following:
Motor
Sensory
Intellectual
Communication
Failure to thrive
Regulatory problems
Failure to thrive
Substance exposure
Developmental
Self-care
Criterion 2.4: A rating of 3 on at least one of the following
School behavior
Social behavior
Sexually reactive behavior
Criterion 2.5: A rating of 2 or 3 on at least one of the following
Suicide risk
Self-mutilation
Other self-harm
Danger to others
Runaway
Sexual aggression
Fire setting
Delinquency

(continued)

Table 5.7 (continued)

A child is suggested for Specialized Foster, if he or she meets EITHER
(a) Criteria 2.1 for referral to Medically Complex OR
(b) Criteria 2.2 and (EITHER 2.3 OR 2.4 OR 2.5) for Mental Health
NOTE: Unless a youth is 15 years old or older and Attachment is rated as a 2 or 3, then consider Group Home (see Group Home criteria below)

Option 3. Group Home/treatment Group Home
For this level three different threshold models should be used, depending on the age of the child
For Children less than 12 years old
Criterion 3a.1: At least one or more 3 or two or more 2 among the following needs
Psychosis
Attention deficit/impulse
Depression
Anxiety
Oppositional behavior
Antisocial behavior
Attachment
Adjustment to trauma
Substance use
Anger control
Affect dysregulation
Eating disturbance
Behavioral regression
Criterion 3a.2: A rating of at least 2 on developmental
Criterion 3a.3: One 3 among the following risk behaviors
Suicide risk
Self-mutilation
Other self-harm
Danger to others
Sexual aggression
Fire setting
Delinquency
Criterion 3a.4: Two or more 2 among the following risk behaviors
Suicide risk
Self-mutilation
Other self-harm
Danger to others
Runaway
Sexual aggression
Fire setting
Delinquency
A child who is less than 12 to be suggested for Group Home, if he or she meets (EITHER Criterion 3a.1 OR Criterion 3a.2) AND (Criterion 3a.3 OR Criterion 3a.4)
- If Criterion 3a.2 is met consider a specialty program
- If sexual aggression is rated a 2 or 3 consider a specialty program
- If physical/medical is rated a 2 or 3 consider a specialty program
- If delinquency is rated a 2 or 3 consider a specialty program

(continued)

Table 5.7 (continued)

For youth ages 12 to 14 years of age:

Criterion 3b.1: At least one or more 3 or two or more 2 among the following needs

- Psychosis
- Attention deficit/impulse
- Depression
- Anxiety
- Oppositional behavior
- Antisocial behavior
- Attachment
- Adjustment to trauma
- Substance use
- Anger control
- Affect dysregulation
- Eating disturbance
- Behavioral regression
- Somatization

Criterion 3b.2: A rating of 2 or 3 on developmental

Criterion 3b.3: One 3 among the following risk behaviors

- Danger to self
- Self-mutilation
- Other self-harm
- Danger to others
- Sexual aggression
- Fire setting
- Delinquency
- Sexually reactive behavior

Criterion 3b.4: Two or more 2 among the following risk behaviors

- Danger to self
- Self-mutilation
- Other self-harm
- Danger to others
- Runaway
- Sexual aggression
- Fire setting
- Delinquency
- Sexually reactive behavior

A 12- to 14-year-old youth would be suggested for Group Home if he or she met (EITHER Criterion 3b.1 OR Criterion 3b.2) AND (EITHER Criterion 3b.3 OR Criterion 3b.4)

- If Criterion 3b.2 is met consider a specialty program
- If sexual aggression is rated a 2 or 3 consider a specialty program
- If physical/medical is rated a 2 or 3 consider a specialty program
- If delinquency is rated a 2 or 3 consider a specialty program

Youth 15 years and older:

Criterion 3c.1: Attachment is rated as a 2 or 3

Criterion 3c.2: Meets criteria for Specialized Foster Care

Criterion 3c.3: Female ward who is pregnant (rated a 2 or 3 on Parenting Role)

(continued)

Table 5.7 (continued)

A youth 15 years or older would be suggested for Group Home if he or she met criteria set for 12 to 14 year olds OR youth met (both Criterion 3c.1 AND Criterion 3c.2) OR youth meets Criterion 3c.3

- If Criterion 3c.2 is met consider a specialty program
- If sexual aggression is rated a 2 or 3 consider a specialty program
- If physical/medical is rated a 2 or 3 consider a specialty program
- If Delinquency is rated a 2 or 3 consider a specialty program
- If Criterion 3c.3 is met consider a specialty program

Option 4. Residential treatment center

Criterion 4.1: At least two or more 3 among the following needs

Psychosis
Attention deficit/Impulse
Depression
Anxiety
Oppositional behavior
Antisocial behavior
Attachment
Adjustment to trauma
Substance use
Anger control
Affect dysregulation
Eating disturbance
Behavioral regression
Somatization

Criterion 4.2: Three or more 2 among the following needs

Psychosis
Attention deficit/impulse
Depression
Anxiety
Oppositional behavior
Antisocial behavior
Attachment
Adjustment to trauma
Substance use
Anger control
Affect dysregulation
Eating disturbance
Behavioral regression
Somatization

Criterion 4.3: A rating of 2 or 3 on developmental

Criterion 4.4: At least one 3 among the following risk behaviors

Suicide risk
Self-mutilation
Other self-harm
Danger to others
Sexual aggression

(continued)

Table 5.7 (continued)

Fire setting
Delinquency
Criterion 4.5: Three or more 2 among the following risk behaviors
Suicide risk
Self-mutilation
Other self-harm
Danger to others
Runaway
Sexual aggression
Fire setting
Delinquency
Judgment
Social behavior
Sexually reactive behavior
To be suggested for RTC, a child should meet (EITHER Criteria 4.1 OR 4.2 OR 4.3) AND (Criteria 4.4 OR 4.5)

- If Criterion 4.3 is met consider a specialty program
- If sexual aggression is rated a 2 or 3 consider a specialty program
- If physical/medical is rated a 2 or 3 consider a specialty program
- If delinquency is rated a 2 or 3 consider a specialty program

Option 5. Transitional living

Criterion 5.1: Youth is 17–19 years old
Criterion 5.2: Youth is 19–21 years old
Criterion 5.3: A rating of 2 or 3 on Independent Living Skills
Criterion 5.4: A rating of 2 or 3 on any of the following
Intimate relations
Parenting role
Victimization
Medication compliance
Criterion 5.5: A rating of 1 higher on Educational Attainment and has not graduated from high school
Criterion 5.6: Does not meet criteria for Group Home or residential treatment
Criterion 5.7: Youth is NOT currently living in a stable foster home
A youth would be suggested for
Level 1 Transitional Living if he or she meets Criterion 5.1 and 5.3 and 5.6 and 5.7
Level 2 Transitional Living if he or she meets Criterion 5.1 and (Criterion 5.3 AND Criterion 5.4) and Criterion 5.6 and 5.7
Level 3 Transitional Living if he or she meets Criterion 5.2 AND (Criterion 5.3 AND Criterion 5.5) and Criterion 5.6 and 5.7

Option 6. Independent living

Criterion 6.1: Youth is 19 years or older
Criterion 6.2: A rating of 0 o 1 on independent living skills
Criterion 6.3: Youth does not meet criteria for Group Home or residential treatment
Criterion 6.4: Youth is NOT currently living in a stable foster home
A youth is suggested for Independent Living if he or she meets Criterion 6.1 AND Criterion 6.2 AND Criterion 6.3 AND Criterion 6.4

than recommended, and some at higher. Comparing placement duration (i.e., stability), among the three groups (matched, lower, or higher), a statistically significant differences is observed ($F(2, 1{,}017) = 3.74$, $p = 0.024$):

- Children placed at higher level than CANS recommended 151.8 days ($n = 240$)
- Children placed at the CANS recommended level 164.8 days ($n = 471$)
- Children placed at a lower level than CANS recommended 134.6 days ($n = 309$)

Figure 5.3 presents a survival curve for placement stability following a CAYIT. The most stable placements are those consistent with the CANS recommendation (match = 0), followed by those who are placed at a less intensive level of care. The least stable placements are those in which the child/youth is placed at a lower level of care than indicated by the CANS (match = 1).

When child family teams following the CANS recommended, the following placement was more stable than if they did not.

Crisis intervention and psychiatric hospitalization

Decision support models also have been used to model decision making about psychiatric hospitalization for children and youth. Initially, we used logistic regression

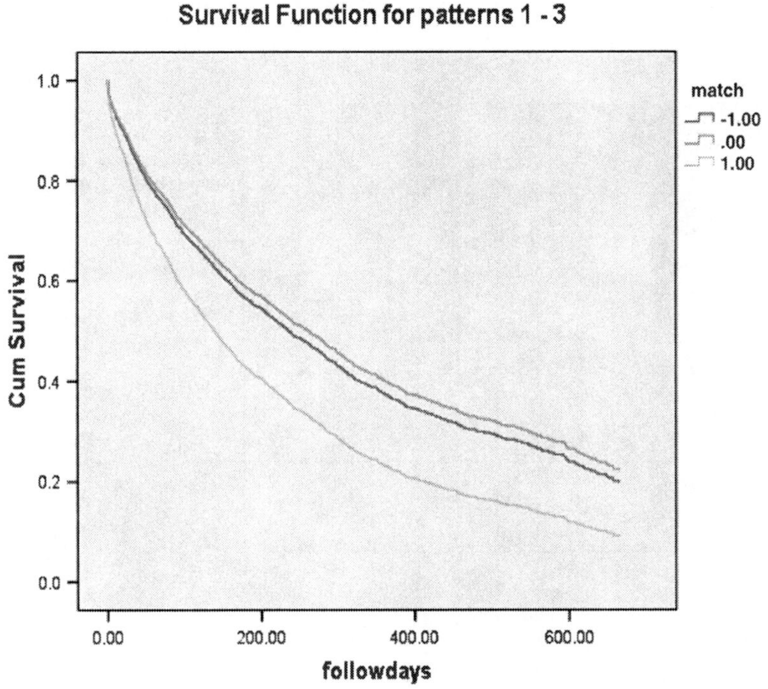

Survival Function for patterns 1 - 3

match
-1.00
.00
1.00

Cum Survival: 1.0, 0.8, 0.6, 0.4, 0.2, 0.0

followdays: 0.00, 200.00, 400.00, 600.00

Figure 5.3 Survival analysis of time to placement disruption for children/youth whose placement matches CANS recommendations (Match = 0), those whose placed is at a lower intensity than recommended (match = −1), and those whose placement is more intensive than recommended (match = 1)

to predict which children/youth would be hospitalized versus served in the community. As evidence mounted we realized that you could not use logistic regression in the field, so we used a log linear model that successfully predicted about 85% of decisions to admit or treat in the community. The model worked used the following indicators adding one point for the presence of each:

- Suicide risk rating of 2 or 3
- Judgment rating of 2 or 3
- Depression rating of 2 or 3
- Impulsivity rating of 2 or 3
- Danger to others rating of 2 or 3
- Anger control rating of 3
- Psychosis rating of 1, 2, or 3

This model results in an indicator that can range from 0 for a child or youth with none of these needs, to a 7 for a child or youth with all of them. Using a sample of 330 crisis episodes we divided the cases into low risk (0 or 1 on the indicator), medium risk (2, 3, or 4 on the indicator), and high risk (5, 6, or 7) on the indicator. Changes on the CSPI total score can be seen over the course of the 90-day crisis episode in Figure 5.4. Review of these findings reveal that psychiatric hospitalization has significantly better outcomes than community treatment for high-risk children/youth, but is associated with reliable worsening for low-risk children/youth.

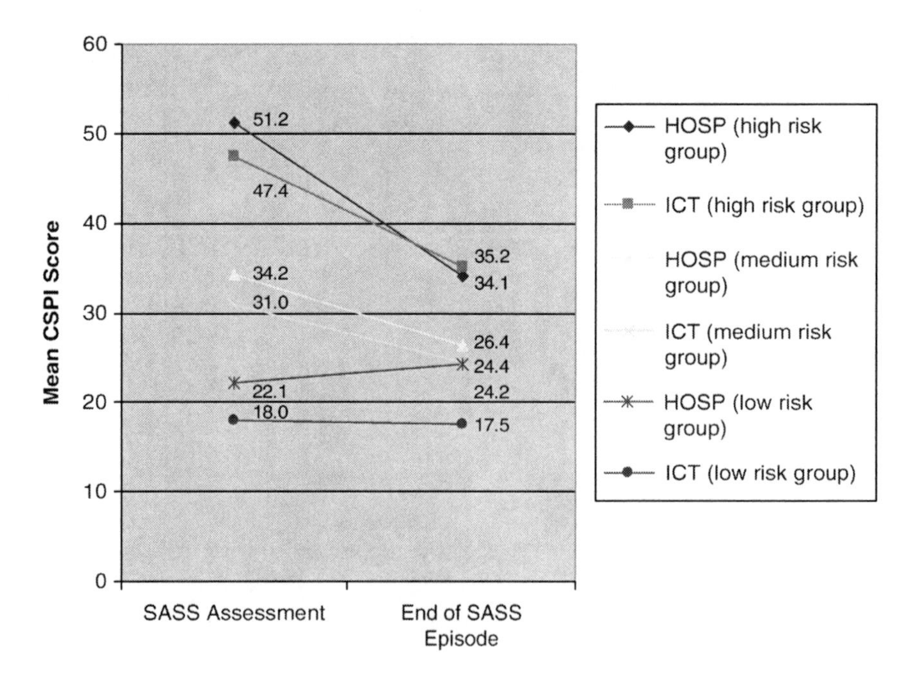

Figure 5.4 Change in total CSPI score by intervention and hospitalization risk level (FY06)

Using CANS Scores to Assess Change Overtime: Outcome Applications

Perhaps the area of greatest controversy with communimetric tools is their suitability to measure change. Anyone who has studied measurement knows that items with restricted options, therefore, have restricted ranges and, de facto, are less sensitive to change than a measure with many options. Of course, anyone who is sophisticated in their knowledge of measuring change also knows that the utility of a measure to assess change is not solely determined by its response options, but also by its reliability and relevance to things that might be expected to actually change. A highly reliable measure can be sensitive to change even when the response options are restricted. An unreliable measure will not be sensitive to detecting real change even with a very large range of scores.

The Childhood Functional Assessment Form is a good example of a measure that fits traditional psychometric theory in terms of allowing a wide range of response options, but whose reliability is so poor that it is not a good measure of change. The CFARS utilizes 10 levels of ratings for each of 16 items.

1. No problem
2. Less than slight
3. Slight
4. Slight to moderate
5. Moderate
6. Moderate to severe
7. Severe
8. Severe to extreme
9. Extreme

Good luck trying to define the actual, meaningful difference between "Slight" and "Less than slight" in actual practice.

Unlike psychometric measures in which clinical significance is a more rigorous standard than statistical significance, any change on the CANS is clinically significant. The child/youth is different in terms of actionable needs. Ironically, statistical significance is actually a more conservative standard and becomes relevant for dimension score analyses. With psychometric tools, statistical significance is generally viewed as a less conservative standard. Reliable change indices have been created for the CANS and the percent of children and youth who demonstrate reliable change (usually a 2–4 point change on the 30-point dimension scale) can be reported. Benchmarks of reliable change for the overall score, individual dimension scores, or the likelihood of any reliable change across all dimensions are available.

As described in scoring options, the CANS can be used for outcomes in two ways. First, the percent change in actionable ratings (or in any levels of ratings) can be studied for individual items. Figure 5.5 demonstrates this type of analysis for behavioral/emotional needs from a wraparound program in New Jersey. Youth with actionable trauma problems account for 26% of all cases at enrollment but by the end of the treatment episode only 16% still have actionable needs regarding Adjustment to Trauma.

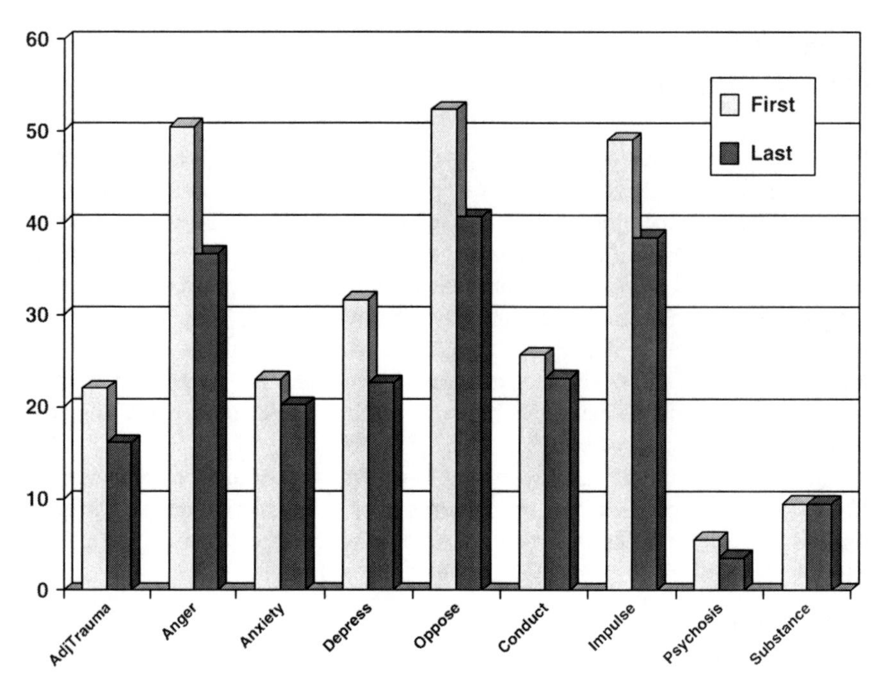

Figure 5.5 New Jersey youth in wraparound services (Care Management Organizations) Percent actionable first and last: Behavioral/Emotional Needs

Outcomes also can be studied with the CANS using dimension scores. This approach is nearly identical to the applications with psychometric measures and should follow the same standards. Concepts such as reliable change and internal consistency of the dimension score are all relevant to the science of outcomes analysis.

Using the CANS dimension scores over time it is possible to track change in residential treatment. Comparisons can be made between youth placed in residential treatment consistent with the CANS recommendation (Concordant) and those placed in residential treatment when the CANS suggested a lower level of care intensity. Figure 5.6 presents the outcome comparison between these two groups for changes in behavioral/emotional needs based on nearly 400 youth. Review of these data indicates that the concordant youth improve over time in residential treatment from their status in the community prior to placement, while the discordant group actually demonstrates a higher level of symptomatology after placement. Figure 5.7 displays the same information for high-risk behaviors. All differences in both figures are statistically significant among groups and over time. These two figures together demonstrate that the reliable worsening observed in the discordant group on behavioral/emotional needs is not a regression to the mean phenomenon, as both groups improved on high-risk behaviors.

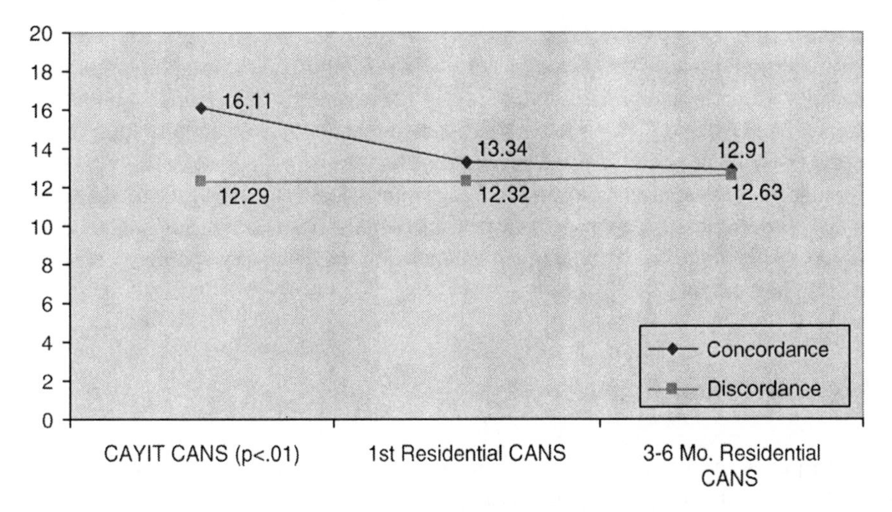

Figure 5.6 Comparison of emotional/behavioral needs between CANS/CAYIT agreed placements in residential treatment (Concordant) and CANS referrals to lower levels of care—children who were placed in residential treatment (Discordant)

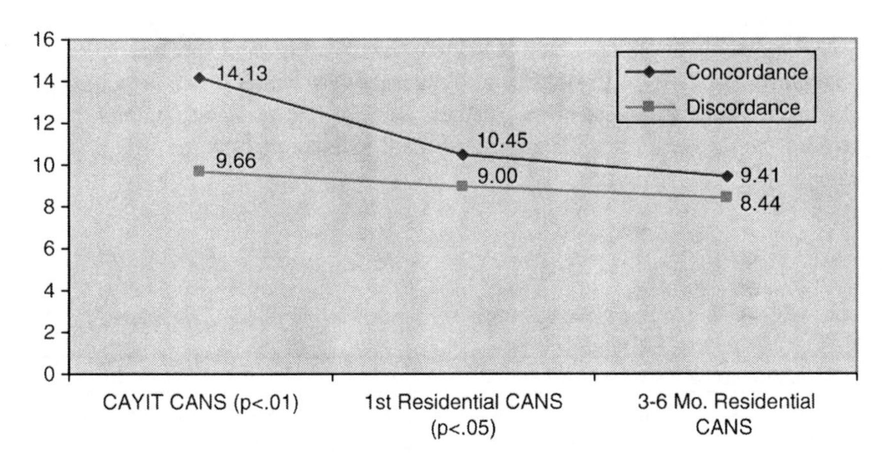

Figure 5.7 Comparison of high-risk behaviors between CANS/CAYIT agreed placements in residential treatment (Concordant) and CANS referrals to lower levels of care—children who were placed in residential treatment (Discordant)

Percent Change Analyses

There is one commonly used type of analysis that is not recommended for CANS or other communimetric tools. Because differences in baseline values with psychometric measures are common and since these measures are by their nature arbitrary, some investigators recommend the use of percent change as a strategy to assess the size of an outcome (Harris, 1967), although others warn against this approach of any outcome analysis (Vickers, 2001). Such analyses are an extremely bad idea with a communimetric tool since the level of the score has a meaning in terms of the intensity or complexity of service needs (or strengths-based opportunities). A change from a 15 to a 10 on a CANS dimension score is substantially more meaningful in terms of need (or strength) than a change from a 3 to a 2. To value these two outcomes as identical, as a percent change model does is forgetting the fundamentals of the communimetric approach. In fact, movement from dangerous and disabling to actionable may be of greater value than moving from actionable to watchful waiting/prevention.

Implementation Experiences

As discussed in Chap. 3, implementation of a communimetric tool is more than just ensuring people complete it. The idea is to fully embed the tool into the fabric of the work where it is being employed. Since the CANS is the first and most evolved communimetric tool, we have substantial experience on its implementation across a broad range of jurisdictions, as demonstrated in Figure 5.1. All of these have been initiated since 2000.

Any statewide implementation is likely to involve requiring specific individuals to complete the CANS. Establishing the methods by which this is accomplished actually becomes an aspect of the business rules of that service system. Table 5.8 provides the business rules for the use of the CANS throughout the Illinois DCFS system.

Table 5.8 CANS assessment business rules for use within the Illinois DCFS system. CANS assessment for administrative case review

1. Person responsible for completing the CANS	
1.1 DCFS/POS caseworker	In all cases, it is the DCFS or POS caseworker's (or the caseworker's supervisor, especially if the current caseworker has been assigned to the case for less than 30 days) responsibility to ensure that a "current" CANS assessment (see definition in 2.1, below) is included in the Administrative Case Review (ACR). This CANS assessment should be completed in the context of the Child and Family Team (CFT) meeting occurring prior to the ACR review. At the time of the CFT meeting, the worker should assemble (contradicted below 2.1 where option is given to complete CANS prior to CFT) all those individuals who have completed a CANS assessment on the youth, or in their absence, should obtain copies of those previously completed CANS. These individuals may include outpatient counselors, therapists, CAYIT reviewers, clinical screeners, SOC workers, or residential staff. As always, the CFT should also include the parents, client, caseworker, and clinical supervisor.

(continued)

Table 5.8 (continued)

1.2 Outpatient behavioral health care provider	Outpatient therapists and counselors may complete the CANS assessment in the course of monitoring progress in outpatient treatment. It is recommended that the CANS be completed every 6 months, and these CANS should be submitted to the caseworker for inclusion in the CFT meeting, during which discussion will take place incorporating all of the supporting documentation into a summary CANS. If the therapist's CANS is the most recent CANS (completed in the last 90 days) and there has been no CAYIT or psychiatric hospitalization, the worker will review the therapist's CANS and use it as the basis for the completion of the CANS that will be submitted to ACR.
1.3 Residential treatment staff	The CANS is completed every 3 months by residential staff. The most recent CANS should be submitted to the worker for inclusion in the CFT discussion regarding the most current CANS. The residential CANS is likely to be the most recent in cases in which there have been no recent CAYIT or psychiatric hospitalizations. In these cases, the residential CANS can be used as the basis for the CANS that will be submitted to ACR. The worker will lead a review of the document in the CFT meeting preceding ACR, at which time item scores will be confirmed by participants and additional information (if available) will be incorporated.
1.4 Integrated assessment clinical screeners	A CANS is completed as part of Integrated Assessment (IA) within the first 45 days of the case. This is most likely to be the child and family's first CANS. Consequently, every effort should be made to collect comprehensive information about the child's history, functioning, strengths, and symptoms. In the IA context, the CANS is used to develop a service plan that targets areas of need and builds upon strengths. The CANS (specifically, the Caregiver Needs and Parent Readiness for Reunification modules) is also used at IA to provide support for permanency goals. If the IA CANS is the only CANS completed in a case thus far, it can be used as a basis for re-scoring at the CFT by the caseworker and team members.
1.5 CAYIT reviewers	A CANS is completed as part of every Child and Adolescent Youth Investment Team (CAYIT) meeting. These meetings evaluate child functioning and appropriateness for placement at times when the placement is in question and a new placement is needed. Although the CAYIT CANS should be submitted to the worker for inclusion in the CFT meeting prior to ACR, if it is the only CANS completed within the last 90 days a new CANS should be completed. In the context of CAYIT the CANS is used to guide decisions about level of care and placement.
1.6 SOC CANS	If the child is receiving SOC services he or she is assessed using the CANS at the initiation of these services and subsequently every 6 months. The SOC CANS should be submitted to the worker for inclusion in the CFT prior to ACR, and if it was completed within 90 days of this meeting it can be used as the basis for the "current" CANS. The SOC CANS is used to develop individualize plans of care for wards that address needs and build upon strengths.

(continued)

Table 5.8 (continued)

2. Principles for determining the "current" CANS	
2.1 Prior to administrative case review	If previously completed CANS (by those individuals mentioned in 1, above, excluding CAYIT or Psychiatric Hospitalization, see below) were completed within 90 days of the CFT prior to ACR, the recent CANS need only be reviewed by the caseworker and item scores confirmed. The caseworker may choose to accept all item ratings, or raise items for revision in the meeting rating areas that have undergone change since the recent CANS was completed. If the previously completed CANS is older than 90 days, the worker must lead the process of completing a CANS assessment, prior to or as part of the CFT meeting. If the caseworker determines that there is no "current" CANS according to these guidelines, a new CANS must be completed. This may require completing the entire document, or, if there is an existing (outdated) CANS, it is acceptable for the DCFS caseworker to review it and use it as the basis for a new CANS in which items that have changed are revised, but existing ratings are maintained in areas in which there has been no change. It is the DCFS caseworker's responsibility to determine whether there is a current CANS, and to initiate the completion of a new one if necessary. Once the CANS has been reviewed, participants in the meeting will sign the document. These participants may include (but are not limited to) the Parents, Client, Caseworker, Therapist, and Clinical Supervisor.
2.2 Under circumstances of psychiatric hospitalization	A current CANS must be reviewed at discharge from the hospital to identify areas of need. The CANS used for discharge planning must be "current" within 3 months. For children who are flagged (those who have been readmitted to the hospital within 30 days of a prior hospitalization, those who are 6 or under, those who are without placement, and those who have been hospitalized 3 or more times in 6 months), a CANS within the last 30 days is required for treatment planning at discharge. For children who have multiple instances of a "flag" trigger, the CANS must be reviewed for treatment planning at discharge but should not be completed more than once in a 30-day period. If the caseworker determines that there is no "current" CANS according to these guidelines, a new CANS must be completed prior to discharge. This may require completing the entire document. Or, if there is an existing (outdated) CANS, it is acceptable for the DCFS caseworker to review it and use it as the basis for a new CANS in which items that have changed are revised, but existing ratings are maintained in areas where there has been no change. It is the DCFS caseworker's responsibility to determine whether there is a current CANS, and to complete a new one if necessary, and bring it to the clinical staffing for review by the DCFS & POS clinical supervisor and the hospital staff. Once the CANS has been reviewed, participants in the meeting will sign the document. These participants may include (but are not limited to) the Physician, Hospital Social Worker, Caseworker, and Clinical Supervisor.

(continued)

Table 5.8 (continued)

3. Procedures for CANS review in CFT meeting	
3.1 Completion of CANS in CFT meeting	Although the caseworker has the ultimate responsibility for completion of the CANS to be included in ACR, the CANS is intended to represent consensus among all of the participants in the CFT meeting. Negotiation among participants on item scores is to be expected and encouraged, as it is only by incorporating all available perspectives on the child's functioning and strengths that the tool can accurately reflect the child's current state.
3.2 Parent readiness for reunification	As long as the goal continues to be "return home," the "Parent Readiness for Reunification" module of the CANS must be completed as part of any CANS administration. This module, comprised of items 101–142, rates the parent's ability to adequately care for the child.
3.3 Transition to adulthood	This section should be completed for all youth in ILO/TLP placements, as well as all youth 14.5 years old. These items are optional in other cases in which the worker deems them appropriate.
4. Training	
4.1 Training	All caseworkers completing the CANS must be trained and certified in its use. DCFS is responsible for providing training opportunities. All caseworkers completing the CANS must obtain recertification each year by completing a case vignette and submitting it for scoring. Certification is contingent upon 70% reliability on scored items.

Matching Child Needs to Specific Providers

A unique aspect of use for the CANS in the DCFS system is the provider database that was launched in April, 2008. This system takes CANS assessment information and matches it to available providers using geomapping technology. For example, if a child has trauma-related treatment needs as identified by the CANS, then providers in their area would be identified by geographic distance. Figure 5.8 presents a screen from this system that identifies the actionable CANS needs and the possible service providers.

By clicking on the identified provider, the caseworker can get directions to the site (Fig. 5.9). In addition, the system gives detailed information about service/treatment options, information needed at intake, special services (e.g., language, day care). Thus, the system is designed to facilitate the full use of the CANS by the DCFS caseworker by making their job more effective and efficient. In the communimetric theory of measurement, this is one of the essential ways that you facilitate the reliability and validity of the measurement process.

Once the system is useful to caseworker in their work with individual children, the same information can be used at the system level for other applications. Figures 5.10 to 5.12 represent a gap analysis. Figure 5.10 is the location of all youth with an actionable substance use problem. Figure 5.11 is a map of the location of every provider in the state who is willing to serve Medicaid-funded youth who have substance use problems. Figure 5.12 then is the overlay of the prior to figures and provides the gap analysis.

Occasion	IA	CAYIT	Residential	Outpatient therapy	ACR	Hospital discharge	SOC
Person responsible for completing the CANS	IA clinical screener	CAYIT reviewer	Residential caseworker	Therapist	Caseworker	Caseworker	SOC Caseworker
Interval	45 days into case	At placement change	At intake, every 3 months, at discharge	Every 6 months	Every 6 months	At discharge	At initiation of SOC, every 6 months, at discharge
Old CANS used if current within	—	—	Current CANS within 3 months	Current CANS within 6 months	Current CANS within 90 days	Current CANS within 90 days (30 days for cases with "triggers"*)	Current CANS within 6 months
Function	Drives the initial service plan by targeting needs and building upon strengths	Used to guide decisions about level of care and placement	Drives treatment plan and interventions	Drives treatment plans and monitors progress in outpatient treatment	Monitors progress of child and family	Current CANS must be reviewed at discharge from the hospital to identify areas of need for services and placement	Used to develop individualized plans of care that address needs and build upon strengths
Sharing	Must be shared with the caseworker and all service providers	Must be shared with the caseworker, residential staff, and service providers	Must be shared with the caseworker and all service providers	Must be shared with the caseworker	Must be shared with all participants in the CFT	Must be shared with all participants in the discharge meeting	Must be shared with the caseworker and service providers

Rule	A new CANS must be completed by the caseworker at 6 months in conjunction with the CFT	If CAYIT CANS is the only CANS completed within the last 90 days a new CANS should be completed by the caseworker in conjunction with the CFT.	The residential CANS is likely to be the most recent in cases where there have been no recent CAYIT or psychiatric hospitalizations. In these cases, the residential CANS can be used as the basis for the CANS that will be submitted to ACR.	If the therapist's CANS was completed within 90 days and there has been no CAYIT or psychiatric hospitalization, the therapist's CANS can be used as the basis for the CANS that will be submitted to ACR.	If Residential, SOC, or a Therapists CANS is the most recent (completed in the last 90 days) (excluding CAYIT or Psychiatric Hospitalization), that CANS can be used as the basis for the CANS that will be submitted to ACR. If the previously completed CANS is older than 90 days, the worker must complete a new CANS.	Any CANS completed within the last 90 days can be considered as a basis for completion of a new CANS upon discharg. This revised CANS must be brought to the clinical staffing with DCFS/POS clinical supervisor and hospital staff.	If the SOC workers CANS is the most recent CANS (completed in the last 90 days) and there has been no CAYIT or psychiatric hospitalization, the worker will review the therapist's CANS and use it as the basis for the completion of the CANS that will be submitted to ACR.

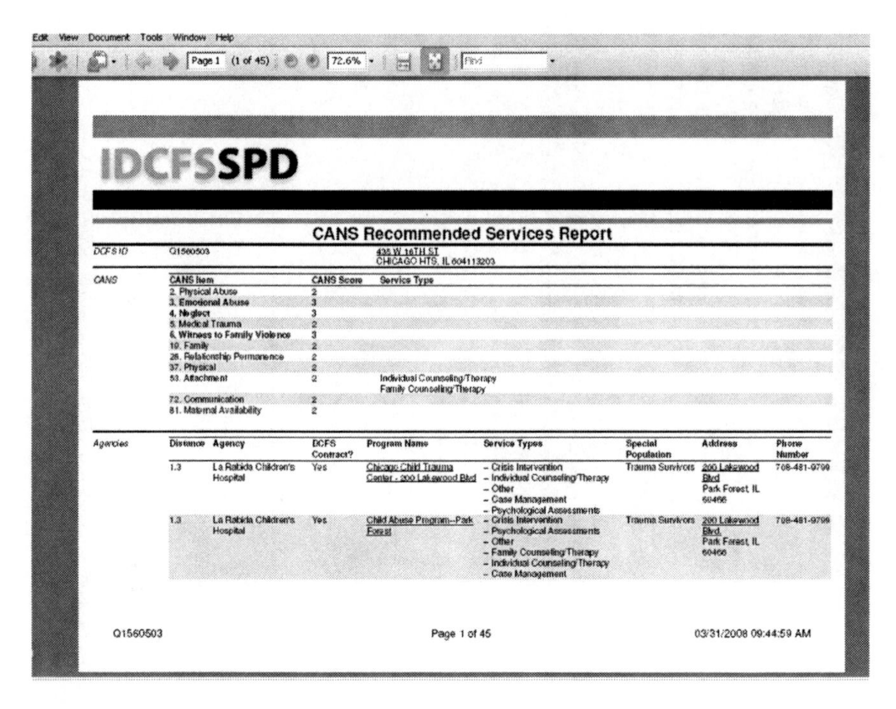

IDCFSSPD

CANS Recommended Services Report

DCFS ID: Q1560503 — 435 W 16TH ST, CHICAGO HTS, IL 604113203

CANS

CANS Item	CANS Score	Service Type
2. Physical Abuse	2	
3. Emotional Abuse	3	
4. Neglect	3	
5. Medical Trauma	2	
6. Witness to Family Violence	3	
19. Family	2	
28. Relationship Permanence	2	
37. Physical	2	
53. Attachment	2	Individual Counseling/Therapy Family Counseling/Therapy
72. Communication	2	
81. Maternal Availability	2	

Agencies

Distance	Agency	DCFS Contract?	Program Name	Service Types	Special Population	Address	Phone Number
1.3	La Rabida Children's Hospital	Yes	Chicago Child Trauma Center - 200 Lakewood Blvd	– Crisis Intervention – Individual Counseling/Therapy – Other – Case Management – Psychological Assessments	Trauma Survivors	200 Lakewood Blvd Park Forest IL 60466	708-481-9799
1.3	La Rabida Children's Hospital	Yes	Child Abuse Program--Park Forest	– Crisis Intervention – Psychological Assessments – Other – Family Counseling/Therapy – Individual Counseling/Therapy – Case Management	Trauma Survivors	200 Lakewood Blvd. Park Forest, IL 60466	708-481-9799

Q1560503 Page 1 of 45 03/31/2008 09:44:59 AM

Figure 5.8 CANS recommended services report

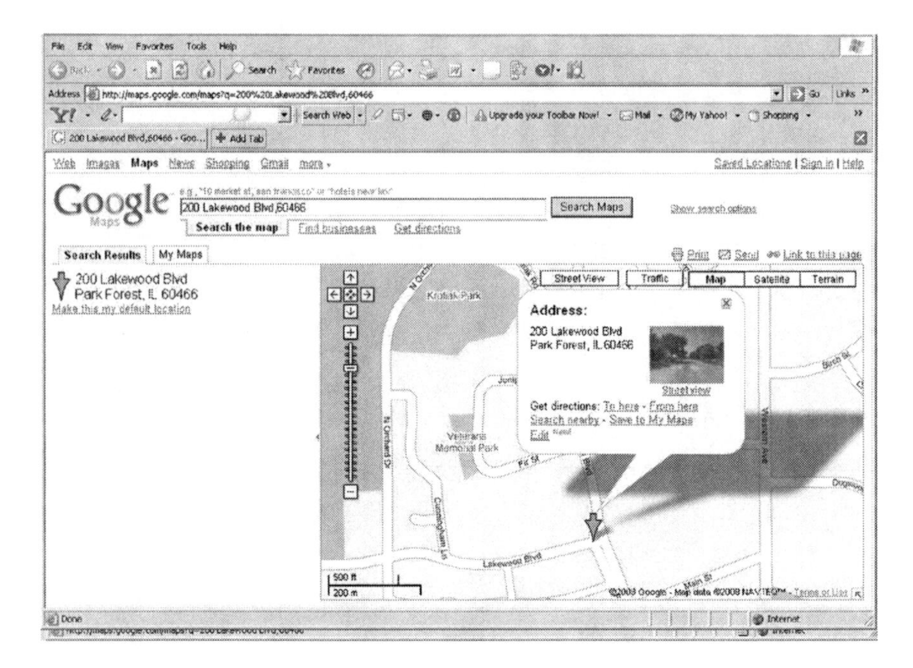

Figure 5.9 Map of all youth with an actionable substance use need in child welfare in Illinois

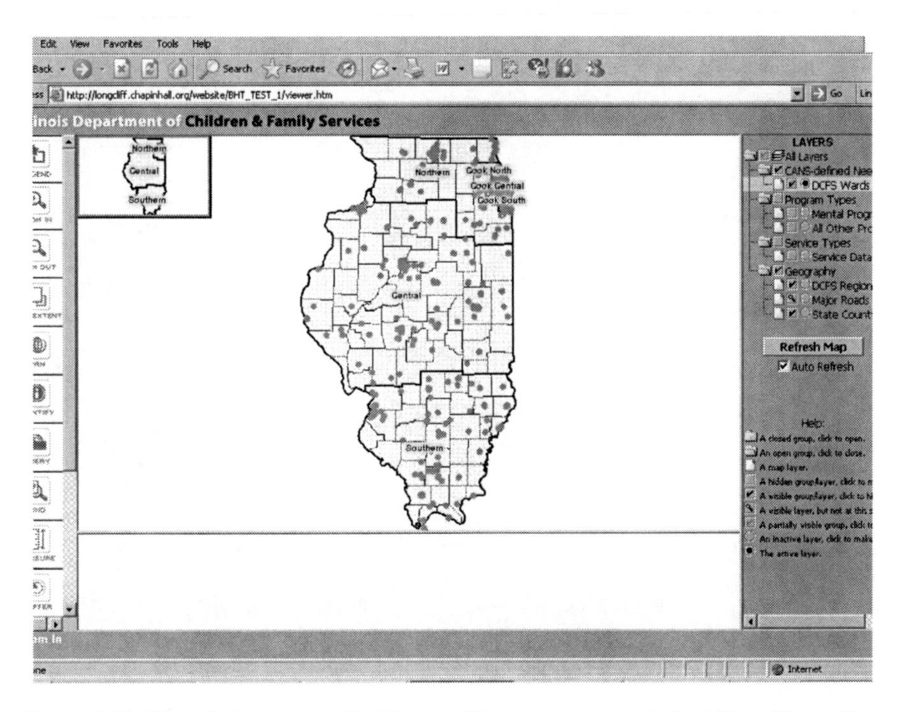

Figure 5.10 Map of all providers in illinois willing to treat a youth in child welfare with a substance use need

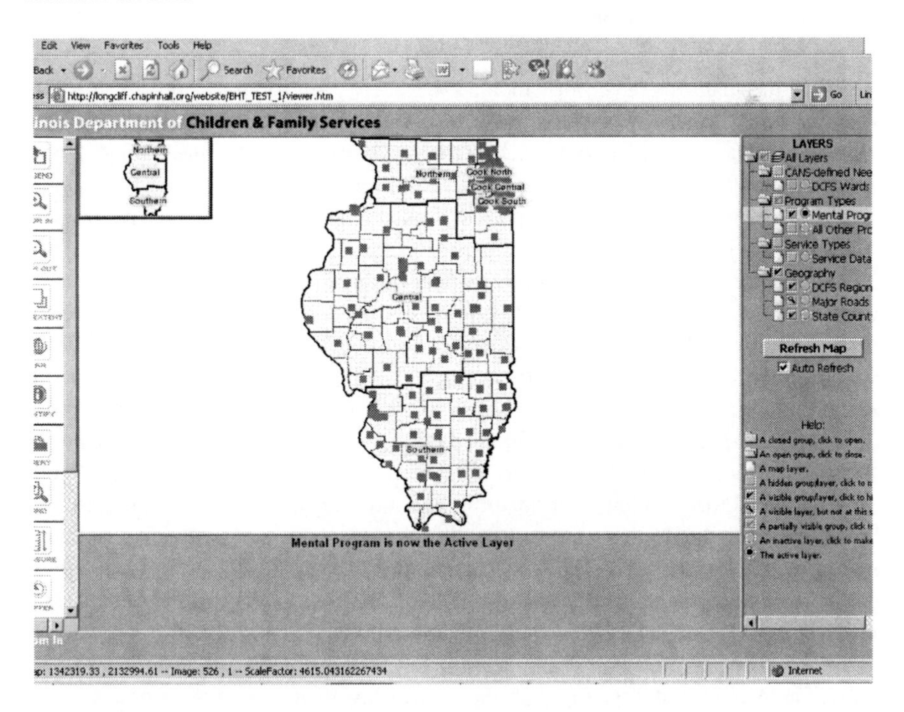

Figure 5.11 Gap analysis comparing youth with needs to the location of providers willing to treat

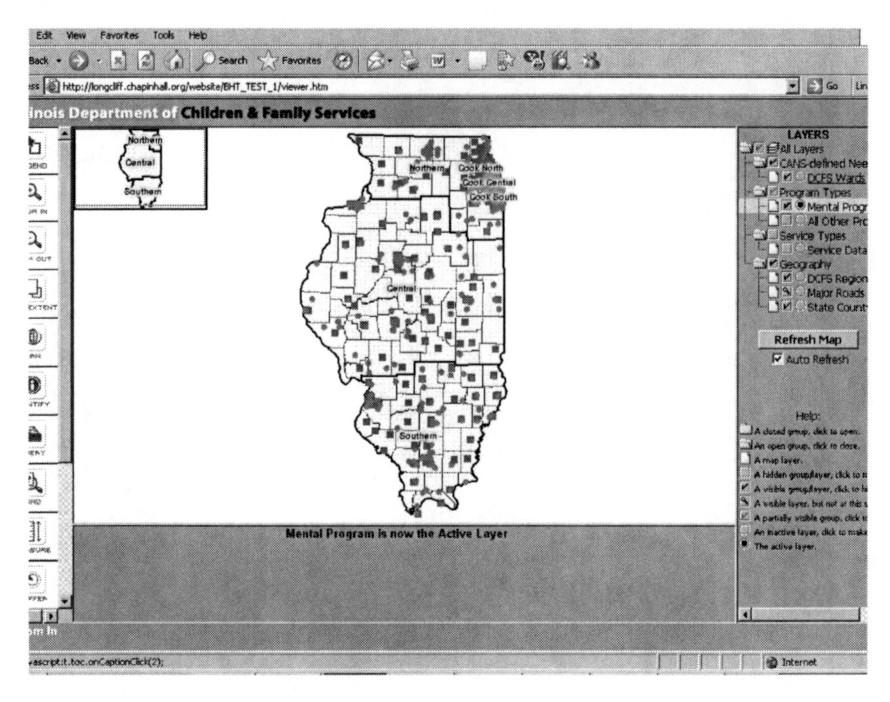

Figure 5.12 Comparison of entry level of needs on the CANS for supportive case management (YCM), intensive community services (CMO) and residential treatment (RTC) over five years of a system of care implementation

Other jurisdictions have implemented the CANS in different ways. New Jersey was the first state to implement the CANS in a cross-systems application. They created two versions of the tool—the Needs Assessment and the Strengths & Needs Assessment—to embed into a new initiative design to create greater access to intensive community services through the creation of Care Management Organizations (CMO) with geographic responsibilities. Referrals to the CMO can come from mental health, juvenile justice, child welfare, or directly from parents who are concerned about their children. The Needs Assessment is used to communicate the needs initially and it is used to determine eligibility for the CMO. Once children are accepted into the program, they receive a full assessment, building on the already identified needs but expand the assessment to include strengths and more details (i.e., modules) about specific needs that are globally identified in the Needs Assessment but require clarification for effective treatment planning. Figure 5.13 presents the admission levels of need on the total score (behavioral/emotional, risk behaviors and functioning) for supportive case management youth case management (YCM), wraparound CMO, and residential treatment (RTC). Review of these comparisons demonstrates that the use of the CANS as a decision support has created a better separation between these dramatically different program types in terms of the needs of the children/youth served. In 2003, there was little difference. By 2007, the average difference among these three levels of care was far greater.

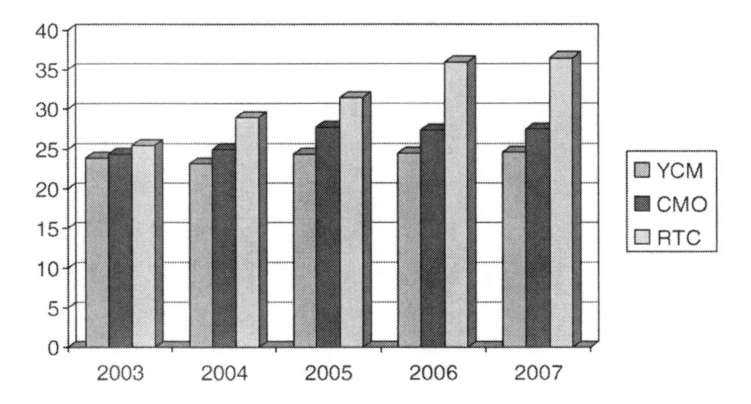

Fig. 5.13 Comparison of total score for RTC, CMO, and YCM initial assessments by year.

Tennessee's Department of Children's Services (DCS) uses the CANS as its initial assessment upon custody. The TN version of the CANS is initiated by the Child Protective Services (CPS) worker based on information collected as part of the investigation. If the child is removed, the CANS assessment process is transferred to a child welfare caseworker to complete. This caseworker builds on the information provided by CPS and completes the CANS in time for the initial child family team, which should take place within about 1 week of the custody decision. The CANS guides placement and permanency planning decisions at that time. The worker then completes the CANS at regular intervals throughout their stay with DCS.

Indiana was the first state to have all four of the major child-serving system partners at the table for the design of their version of the CANS: mental health, child welfare, juvenile justice, and the schools. As a result, they identified and designed a new item, "Bullying," to include this very important need within the school system. Of course, this item was put into the mass collaboration mode (see Chap. 8), and a number of other jurisdictions now have included it in their version. Data from the first year indicate that bullying is the second most common high-risk behavior after "Social Behavior" among children and youth receiving mental health services in the state.

Since 2000, the CANS has become a widely used tool for implementing change in the child-serving system in the United States and elsewhere. Its rapidly spreading popularity alone suggests that it is useful. The emerging data from the various implementations suggest that the application of this approach is actually transforming for the child-serving system to improve efficiency and effectiveness.

Chapter 6
The Intermed

Engel (1977) proposed the breakthrough biopsychosocial model for the practice of medicine. In his classic treatise, he argued that understanding medicine required the physician to conceptualize more than just the disease state. Good medical care requires consideration of psychological and social variables as well. Since that time there have been many innovations for improving treatment for patients with psychological and social complications to their medical condition (e.g., Strain et al., 1991). Strategies from physician education to integrating psychiatric, psychological, and social services into primary, secondary, and tertiary medical care have been described. However, despite the fact that the word *biopsychosocial* has become fully integrated in our lexicon, it has not always been the case that medicine has shifted paradigms from the traditional medical model into a broader model that formally includes the assessment of psychological and social variables that influence treatment decisions and prognosis in health care.

Worldwide, the health care system has changed rapidly over the past two decades. Some of that change has been fostered by advances in medical procedures and technology. Some change has evolved from shifts in investments and funding strategies. Other changes have resulted from cultural shifts about the role of the person in his or her own health care. Still others have resulted from the success of medicine in treating acute illness, leading to an increased prevalence of chronic illness with comorbidities (Druss, 2006). Table 6.1 presents Huyse and Stiefel's (2006) conceptualization regarding the shift from traditional guiding principles (referred to as *rules* by these authors) and the guiding principles that have taken root in postmodern medicine as discussed in the landmark publication *Crossing the Quality Chasm: A New Health System for the 21*st *Century*, by the Institute of Medicine (2001).

Review of this table suggests that the very nature of health care is shifting away from the solo practice of a physician operating alone in his or her community whose autonomy is respected by all parties in the system. In the old model, the physician made all the decisions with regard to diagnosis and treatment. Specialization, the dramatic increase in the knowledge base about human health, and the expansion and growth of allied health professionals make the traditional model based on the office practice of a general practitioner seem quaint. Even direct marketing of new medications to prospective patients affects the role of the physician (Lyles, 2002).

J.S. Lyons, *Communimetrics: A Communication Theory of Measurement in Human Service Settings*,
DOI 10.1007/978-0-387-92822-7_6,

Table 6.1 Evolution of the Guiding Principles That Determine Patient Care

Traditional Guiding Principles	New Guiding Principles
Care is based on visits	Care is based on continuous healing relationships
Professional autonomy drives variability	Care is customized to patient's needs and values
Professionals control care	Patients control care
Information is a record	Knowledge is shared and information flows freely
Decisions are based on training and experience	Decision making is evidence based
"Do not harm" is the responsibility of the clinician	Safety is a system responsibility
Secrecy is necessary	Transparency is necessary
The system reacts to need	Needs are anticipated
Cost containment and reduction is sought	Waste is continuously decreased
Professional identity is preferred over system functioning	Cooperation among clinicians is a priority

Source: Institute of Medicine, 2001.

Further, emerging evidence demonstrates that psychosocial problems among persons with medical illness have a variety of untoward consequences, including poorer health outcomes, diminished quality of life (De Jonge, Ormel, & Slaets, 2004), reduced compliance with treatment (Dimatteo, Lepper, & Croghan, 2000), excessive health care use (Ciechanowski, Katon, & Russo, 2000), and premature death (Wulsin, Vaillant, & Wells, 1999).

These complexities suggest that optimal medical care requires integration across multiple specialists and health care providers. There are a variety of challenges to the collaboration required for integration (San Martin-Rodriguez, Beaulieu, & D'Amour, 2005). For example, in primary care, the time available to a physician when meeting with each patient can be quite limited. Gandhi et al. (2000) reported that nearly two-thirds of primary care doctors were dissatisfied with their communications with specialists. In hospital care, communication among the large number of health professionals working with a single patient can be daunting. While Marshall (1998) reports high levels of cross-discipline and specialty respect, when a patient experiences multiple comorbidities that require the input of different specialists, coordination of different, potentially competing treatment protocols can be challenging even in the best of circumstances. In fact, communication has been described as a significant factor in many medical errors (Elder & Dovey, 2002). Baggs, Ryan, Phelps, Richeson, and Johnson (1992) reported an association between nurse-perceived collaboration and patient outcomes, even controlling for severity of illness. Rowe, Garcia, Macfarlane, and Davidson (2001) report an association between poor communication and the likelihood of stillbirths and infant deaths. Therefore, as health care becomes more complex, the role of communication in health care becomes more important.

Communication problems have been linked to a variety of problems, including poor continuity of care, delayed diagnosis and treatment, polypharmacy, litigation, and redundant testing (Epstein, 1998). There are at least two areas in which communication problems can interfere with effective medical interventions (Dovey, Meyers, & Phillips 2002). First, it has been often observed that patients and health care providers can have different perspectives on the same symptoms and treatments (Slade, Phelan, & Thornicroft, 1998). In fact, efforts to use measurement to facilitate communication between patients and health care professionals have been reported in mental health (van Os et al., 2002, 2004).

The second area of communication that is critical to effective medical intervention is among health professionals. While primary care offices often require only communication between the physician and patient for issues of medical care, other health care settings can be far more complex in terms of the number of different health professionals participating in the medical care of one patient. De Jonge, Huyse, and Steifel (2006) make the distinction between the related concepts of case complexity and care complexity. Case complexity is a characteristic of a patient's presentation. Care complexity is a characteristic of the treatment environment. One central factor that makes care more complex is when multiple health professionals are involved in the treatment of the same patient. Care is complex because it must be coordinated or integrated among professionals involved in the treatment of the patient. Communication among these health professionals is the first step toward at least coordinated care and ultimately integrated care (Wulsin, Sollner, & Pincus, 2006). Existing research suggests that the experience of good communication and collaboration varies across tasks, settings, and disciplines (Beuscart-Zephir, Pelayo, Anxeaux, Maxwell, & Suerlinger, 2007; Larson, Hamilton, Mitchell, & Eisenberg, 1998; Makary et al., 2006; Newton et al., 1994).

Case complexity is related to care complexity. Generally the more complex the case, the more complex the medical care is likely to be. However, this relationship is by no means perfectly linear. For example, various forms of rehabilitation (e.g., cardiac, stroke) might be relatively simple from a case perspective, but somewhat complex in terms of medical care. However, in general, the most complex cases require the greatest amount of communication and coordination in order to achieve effective, integrated medical care.

A variety of approaches have been presented for improving communication in medical care settings. Pronovost et al. (2003) describe the value of using a daily goal list in intensive care that reduced length of stays 50%, from an average of 2.2 days to 1.1. Others have used similar approaches that focus on daily treatment goals (Phipps & Thomas, 2007; Schmidt, Claesson, Westerholm, Nilsson, & Svarstad, 1998). Some have used more team-building types of strategies (e.g., Boyle & Kochinda, 2004; Curley, McEachern, & Speroff, 1998). Still other approaches have utilized information technology (Aarts, Ash, & Berg, 2007; Bal, Mastboom, Spiers, & Rutten, 2007; Sidlow & Katz-Sidlow, 2006).

There have been many attempts to assess the severity of disease. Susan Horn's classic work on the Severity of Illness is a good example (Horn, 1983). Disease staging is another approach that attempt to get at the severity of a medical condition (e.g., WHO, 1990). Efforts to assess complexity have lagged behind. One early effort was simply counting the number of diagnoses another (in the pre-electronic medical record days) was weighing the medical chart. Given the experiences in the European Consultation/Liaison Workgroup (ECLW), a subgroup of interested researchers began to develop a measure of case complexity to inform a biopsychosocial approach to medical care (Huyse, Herzog, Malt, & Lobo, 1996). First, an effort was made to use existing information from hospital databases to construct a measure of case complexity consisting of risk factors for care complexity (De Jonge et al., 2001). The INTERMED was the second effort to assess case complexity and the first to embrace a biopsychosocial perspective (Stiefel et al., 1999).

Development of the INTERMED

The European Consultation/Liaison Work Group was established by Frits Huyse in the Netherlands, Thomas Herzog in Germany, Antonio Lobo in Spain, and Uricht Malt in Norway. This multi-site, transnational collaboration was an effort to better understand the role of C/L Psychiatry in Europe (Huyse et al., 1996). A major thrust of this work was to understand which patients were served by C/L Psychiatry and to what end. In other words, what was the current role for C/L Psychiatry in a medical/surgical hospital setting in Europe, and how do you optimize that role for effective health care?

In the 1980s and 1990s there was a body of work demonstrating that psychiatric comorbidities were complicating factors in the hospital care of medical/surgical patients, both in terms of health outcomes and cost of care (e.g., Fulop, Strain, Vita, Hammer, & Lyons., 1989; Lyons et al., 1988). Psychiatric interventions were developed and tested that involved consultation with other health professionals (Smith, Rost, & Kashner, 1995), or integration into treatment teams using a liaison strategy (Strain et al., 1991). Both of these interventions were reported to be associated with improved patient outcomes and reduced health care costs. At the same time, other research was demonstrating that social factors had a similar impact on health care (cf., House, 2002).

Attempting to screen patients for psychiatric comorbidities proved difficult because of both methodological and practical concerns. Even the gold standard of a clear psychiatric diagnosis in a medical/surgical patient is rather complicated. Also, because of the time constraints and volume of patient care in hospital, it was not likely that a diagnosis-based case finding strategy would be feasible, let alone successful.

Using data from the participating site for the ECLW, De Jonge and colleagues began to develop the concept of complexity as the feature that involved both psychiatric and social complications to health care. In the process of this research, the ongoing consultation vs. liaison debate re-emerged (Huyse & Steifel, 2006) regarding whether C/L Psychiatry served patients with diagnosed or at least diagnosable psychiatric disorders in the hospital or served a broader role in the comprehensive care of patients in these settings. The assessment and management of complexity is clearly not a specialty skill; by definition it must cross all specialties to be effective. Therefore, a focus on complexity requires an assessment strategy that is efficient and reasonably easy to use for a wide variety of health care professionals. Initially the effort was to see whether information that was routinely collected in electronic records could be used to identify complex patients (De Jonge, Huyse & Steifel, 2006). It quickly became clear that reliance on convenience databases, although a standard for health services research, was insufficient to build an optimal model of the complex patient. For this reason, the INTERMED was developed.

Design of the INTERMED

The first step in the development of the INTERMED was to identify the relevant items to be included in this approach. Rather than a focus group approach, as used with the CANS, a conceptual model provided the framework for the selection of items of this tool. Specifically, items were identified by using the biopsychosocial assessment grid first developed by Hoyle Leigh and others at Yale (Leigh, Feinstein, & Reiser, 1980). This grid was widely used for training and supervision in C/L Psychiatry. Items were selected to present each of the cells in this grid, which included medical, psychological, social, and health systems on one axis and historical, current status, and prognosis on the second axis.

Table 6.2 provides a matrix organization of the structure of the INTERMED. The first three rows represent the biopsychosocial model with the essential concepts for biological, psychological, and social aspects of a patient's life that are relevant to his or her health care. A fourth row exists to allow for a simultaneous monitoring of the patient's experience with the health care system. The columns represent how the medical model of care understands time as it relates to patient

Table 6.2 Item Structure of the INTERMED

	History	Current State	Prognosis
Biological	Chronicity	Severity of symptoms	Complications and life threat
	Diagnostic dilemma	Diagnostic challenge	
Psychological	Restrictions in coping	Resistance to treatment	Mental health threat
	Psychiatry dysfunction	Psychiatric symptoms	
Social	Restrictions in integration	Residential instability	Social vulnerability
	Social dysfunction	Restrictions of network	
Health Care	Intensity of treatment	Organization of care	Coordination
	Treatment experience	Appropriateness of referral	

care, with the history setting the background for comprehensive assessment, current status driving the treatment plan within this context, and prognosis establishing considerations for follow-along care.

History

Biological Domain

This domain allows the rater to describe the acuity or chronicity of the patient's medical condition along with any prior episodes of diagnostic uncertainty. The distinction between acute and chronic diseases is thought to be important, particularly among the elderly (Stiefel et al., 2006). Prior challenges with making diagnoses are important to note, as these challenges may inform the current diagnosis.

Psychological Domain

This domain allows the rater to describe both the patient's past challenges with coping and whether he or she has a history of any diagnosed psychiatric disorders. The concept of these items is that by providing a historical context, the health care providers are assisted in understanding any current difficulties that the patient may experience with regard to managing his or her medical condition and treatment.

Social Domain

This domain provides an assessment of the patient's social connectedness in terms of people, leisure activities, and work. These items can be a flag for the involvement of social work, occupational therapy, or recreational therapy intervention. Social support and connectedness are powerful indicators of good outcomes in health care. Social supports also can assist the patient with activities that may be limited because of his or her current illness.

Health Care Domain

Here the rater can describe any problems in the past that the patient has experienced with his or her health care. Both the intensity of any prior treatment and whether the individual had any negative experiences with his or her health care are described. Prior negative experiences with health care can impact an individual's adherence to new medical regimens and prescriptions. Building a strong relationship between the patient and his or her health care providers is important to effective care.

Current State

Biological Domain

When current status is assessed, it involves the patient's current health status. Items include a rating of how severe his or her symptoms are presently. Also, a rating is provided for the complexity of the medical diagnosis. Together, severity and complexity capture the two key characteristics of any disease state as it affects treatment.

Psychological Domain

In the current state, the presence of any symptoms of psychiatric illness are identified in this domain. In addition, emotional or psychological factors related to the patient's struggle with accepting treatment and maintaining adherence to treatment protocols are described. Thus, this cell describes both current psychiatric comorbidities that may require integrated care and the psychological aspects of adjusting to the patient's current medical status.

Social Domain

Current social issues are described in terms of currently having a stable housing situation and supportive others. Both of these constructs have been identified as critical to support community treatment and avoid institutional placements. Severely ill patients can be increasingly managed in the community if provided with significant social support.

Health Care Domain

In this cell, the organizational complexity of care is described in terms of the number and types of health care professionals involved in the current treatment. Also, the appropriateness of any specialty referrals and transitions are described (e.g., premature discharge).

Prognosis

Biological Domain

Most medical conditions have a known prognosis for the trajectory of recovery. This domain allows the rater to describe the patient's medical prognosis in terms of possible complications and risk of premature death.

Psychological Domain

The mental health threat in the future is rated here. This item identifies the need for ongoing mental health follow-up after the current episode of treatment.

Social Domain

Anticipated social needs are described using an item called Social Vulnerability. This item allows the identification of whether the patient's social circumstances place him or her at risk for complications to ongoing medical treatment.

Health Care Domain

The items on this domain allow the rater to indicate the level of ongoing care coordination needs anticipated based on the individuals medical, psychological, and social functioning. The more medical professionals involved with ongoing care, the greater the level of coordination necessary.

Establishing Action Levels

Once the content areas of the INTERMED were identified, the second step was to identify the action levels using four levels. In computerized applications, colors are associated with these four levels (green, yellow, orange, and red, respectively).

0 No vulnerability, no need to act
1 Mild vulnerability and need for monitoring or prevention
2 Moderate vulnerability and need for treatment or inclusion in the treatment plan
3 Severe vulnerability and need for immediate action or intensive treatment

The following are four example items from the INTERMED, one from each domain. For the biological dimension:

Diagnostic challenge:

0 Clear diagnosis
1 Clear differential diagnosis
2 Complex differential diagnosis in which a diagnosis from a biological perspective is to be expected
3 Complex differential diagnosis in which no diagnosis is to be expected from a biological perspective

From the psychological dimension:
Psychiatric dysfunction:

0 No psychiatric dysfunction
1 Psychiatric dysfunction without clear effects on daily functioning
2 Psychiatric dysfunction with clear effects on daily functioning
3 Psychiatric admissions and/or permanent effects on daily functioning

From the social dimension:
Restrictions in network:

0 Good contacts with families, work, and friends.
1 Restrictions in one of the domains
2 Restrictions in two of the domains
3 Restrictions in three of the domains

And, from the health care system
Treatment experience:

0 No problems with health care professionals
1 Negative experience with health care providers (self or relative)
2 Requests for second opinions or changing contacts with doctors
3 Repeated conflicts with doctors or involuntary admissions

Often in complex medical care environments, health professionals other than physicians are involved in information gathering and communication. In hospital settings, nurses have commonly been trained to complete the INTERMED. The process by which the INTERMED is completed is an information integration strategy. First, the health professional reviews the patient's chart to check current status and any documented history. This review provides a grounding so that the open-ended questions can be responded to in a manner that both allows more targeted questioning and communicates to the patient that the interviewer has "done his or her homework" and is not simply forcing him or her to repeat the story again.

To complete the INTERMED, an interview format has been developed that can be used by a nurse, social worker, or physician. Examples of questions from this interview format include the following:

Now, first of all, I would like to better understand how you feel physically.

Have you ever seen a psychiatrist or have there been periods in your life that you have been anxious, depressed, or confused?

Have there been issues with doctors during the last 5 years that gave you a bad feeling to such an extent that it might interfere with your trust in doctors?

Once completed, the INTERMED has a Web-based platform that allows the user to enter ratings and display them in a fashion that promotes patient care management. The use of the four colors—green, yellow, orange, and red—to highlight the action levels of the ratings makes the graphic display of the biopsychosocial grid quite easy to view and rapidly assimilate the information contained in the assessment. A viewer's eyes are drawn to the vivid red and orange dots marking the actionable needs.

Reliability and Validity

There is a substantial amount of published research using the INTERMED across a range of patient populations and health care systems (e.g., Huyse et al., 2001; Stiefel et al., 1999). In addition, the INTERMED has been studied in a number of different languages.

As with all communimetric tools, reliability should be observed at the item level. Huyse et al. (1999) in the first publication on the reliability of this approach report item reliability based on 14 trained observers using a medical chart review method. Both the intraclass and rank correlation estimates of reliability can be found in Table 6.3.

Review of Table 6.3 reveals that most items were reliable well within expected standards. Nearly half of the items had intraclass correlations of 0.90 or higher. Fifteen of the items had reliabilities of 0.80 or above. Only five items did not have adequate reliability. These items were studied and either revised or the training was altered to improve reliability. It is noteworthy that the prognoses section accounted

Table 6.3 Item Level Reliability of the INTERMED

Item	Intraclass	Rank Correlation
History		
Chronicity	0.98	0.79
Diagnostic uncertainty	0.86	0.71
Restrictions in coping	0.94	0.46
Premorbid level of psychiatric dysfunction	0.97	0.92
Family disruption	0.93	0.87
Impairment in social support	0.92	0.84
Intensity of prior treatment	0.98	0.70
Prior treatment experience	0.41	0.60
Current State		
Severity of illness	0.90	0.50
Clarity of diagnostic profile	0.84	0.82
Treatment resistance	0.92	0.84
Severity of psychiatric symptoms	0.62	0.78
Residential instability	0.88	0.58
Impairment in social integration	0.93	0.75
Organization complexity at admission/referral	0.87	0.52
Appropriateness of admission/referral	0.26	0.61
Prognoses		
Complications and life threat	1.00	0.80
Mental health threat	0.49	0.58
Social vulnerability	0.80	0.29
Care needs	0.44	0.41

As reported in Huyse et al., 1999.

Please cite Lenert et al., 2000 and Slade, Phelan, & Thornicroft, 1998 in the references or delete from text.

Please cite De Jonge, 2002 in the references or delete from text.

for most of the unreliable items. This finding led to a retooling of the training and descriptions around the ratings of prognosis. A couple of the items were difficult to score from the chart review method, resulting in lower reliability (e.g., family disruption, appropriateness of referral/admission).

Validity has been studied a number of different ways. Stiefel et al. (1999) report a study whereby a sample of low back pain patients were clustered into three groups using the INTERMED. Their groups demonstrated reliability differences across a series of other measures, including the Hospital Anxiety and Depression Scale (Zigmond & Snaith, 1983), the medical outcome study Short Form 36 (SF-36; McHorney, Ware, & Raczek, 1993; Ware & Sherbourne, 1992), measures of social support (Meyers & Budowski, 1995), and visual analog pain scales (Jaeschke, Singer, & Guyatt, 1990). The clusters were reliably different on both medical data and the psychometric measures used.

Utility validity is demonstrated by the wide set of patient populations for which INTERMED applications have been reported (Huyse & Steifel, 2006). Among these populations are pain patients, general ambulatory care patients, spinal injury patients, diabetes patients, and the fragile elderly. The technology that supports the use of a color coded INTERMED (red for 3, orange for 2, yellow for 1, and green for 0) as a tool during daily rounds furthers the use validity of this approach. The fact that attending physicians, residents, and nursing staff all report positive experiences with this approach is further evidence of its use validity in complex environments. The INTERMED has not been required in any jurisdiction on all patients, so it is not possible to report on use penetration statistics.

Training and Use

The training on the INTERMED is more intensive than that used with the CANS. Generally, 2-day training is used in which the tool is described and reviewed. An interview format is recommended to collect information directly from patients and family, and training is provided in this interview approach as well. As with the CANS, case studies are used to assess reliability and reliability criteria are required to complete training and reach certification in the tool.

In most implementations the INTERMED is completed by a nurse or care coordinator. When this occurs that individual consults with the medical chart and/or the physician as the starting point of the assessment process. They tend to use the interview format to fill in the missing information (generally on the psychological, social, and health care domains). The INTERMED rater then completes the tools and shares the results with the treatment team in rounds, case conference, or through an electronic medical record that is viewable by all team members.

Like any other numerical rating system, the numbers themselves do not stand alone. The INTERMED shares its method with other communimetric tools that ratings of 2 or 3 require text comments to provide the specifics of those actionable needs across the four domains. Thus, if residential stability is rated a 3, then a comment such as, "Patient lost his apartment and has been sleeping on a friend's couch" or some other such detailed description of the housing situation would be provided.

The INTERMED is the second most commonly used communimetric tool following the CANS. It has the widest applications across different cultures, as the tool has been translated into large number of languages and has enjoyed widespread use in Europe. The Case Management Association of America has recently adopted the INTERMED for this use and has initiated implementation among some of its 30,000 members in the United States.

Chapter 7
The Entrepreneurial League System Assessment

Governments need a successful economy. A successful economy is dependent on the success of individual business enterprises and their abilities to converge into a successful marketplace. In democracies, politicians generally require economic stability or growth to ensure re-election. In totalitarian states, a poor economy can be the impetus for a coup. Given this basic truth of governing, local, state, and federal governments have sought to create opportunities for business success. For a significant part of the world economy, a large segment is dominated by a relatively small number of enormous corporations. This trend continues and expands with globalization. Despite these changes, it remains the case that most businesses are actually small businesses. Although large corporations dominate the business news; small businesses are the foundation of a vigorous economy and spread the wealth in a fashion that is challenging for large enterprises. Successful entrepreneurs are the engine of a vital and egalitarian economy driven by successful small business enterprises. Therefore, a flourishing small business sector is a very desirable economic and political outcome (e.g., Sheahan, 2008).

In a completely open and free marketplace, new businesses live and die based on the quality of their business idea and their ability to delivery a product that sells at a price above what it costs to produce. However, there are few if any entirely open and free marketplaces left in the world. Despite free trade agreements among counties (e.g., European Union, North Atlantic Free Trade Agreement), government regulation is commonplace. From rules about hiring and firing, to workplace safety, to product advertisement, to accounting practices, government regulations abound and multiply. When governments intervene it is with the aim of perfecting these imperfect markets. The challenge for government is to intervene without destroying the fundamentals of the marketplace. Creating government dependency is one sure path to market destruction. Therefore, governments often can have an important role in the development of a thriving small business sector, either positive or negative. The question faced by governments then, is how to best create or incubate small businesses to help the good ones be successful without creating government dependency from what would otherwise be a failing business.

The standard assumption in enterprise development is that a lack of capital might prevent a good idea from becoming a successful business (Durr, Lyons, & Lichtenstein, 2000).

J.S. Lyons, *Communimetrics: A Communication Theory of Measurement in Human Service Settings*,
DOI 10.1007/978-0-387-92822-7_7,

Once a business is appropriately capitalized, its success or failure is a function of market forces. Therefore, there are two critical features of a successful business launch: (1) a good idea that fits the marketplace, and (2) sufficient capital to launch it in that market. With that in mind, most jurisdictions approach business development through the use of service provider organizations. Examples of these approaches include entities such as small business assistance centers, business incubators, microenterprise programs, community revolving loans programs, venture and angel capital groups, university small business assistance centers, and local chambers of commerce, among others. They operate by offering a service or range of services to local entrepreneurs. However, consistent with Gilmore and Pine (1997), these approaches provide entrepreneurs with services when starting a business that may require a transformation of the entrepreneur himself or herself (Lichtenstein & Lyons, 2001).

Providing business service support or capital investment may not be sufficient to effectively stimulate a sustainable business startup. Historically, these programs have used business plans to support decisions about capital investment or service support. This allows the investor to estimate the value of the "good idea." The problem with this approach is twofold. First, successful entrepreneurship is a complex construct. A good idea is a necessary condition for the successful entrepreneur, but by no means is it sufficient. Often characteristics of the entrepreneur facilitate his or her success. For example, entrepreneurs must be able to solve problems and not quit after short-term failures. Second, it is easy enough to hire a consultant to come up with a business plan for capital investment. This does not necessarily mean that the entrepreneur even understands the plan, let alone is able to actually implement this business plan once funding is secured.

An alternative model for growing small businesses is one that embraces the concept that developing successful small businesses should be a process of developing small business people (Lichtenstein & Lyons, 2001). Such activities would fall within the purview of what we have been calling human service enterprises—a transformational offering. Identification and development of the talents, skills, and assets of the entrepreneur become a central focus of the business incubation process. Identifying the qualities and skill sets an entrepreneur has and those he or she must develop and then working with them to develop needed skills is the route toward building successful small business enterprises in this model. Lichtenstein and Lyons (2001) have elaborated this model into a tiered system that they call the Entrepreneurial League System. This approach is grounded on three essential assertions:

1. That entrepreneurs achieve success by developing a skill set
2. That entrepreneurial skill can be developed
3. That entrepreneurs come to entrepreneurship at different skill levels

The Entrepreneurial League System Assessment

Among major sports, baseball is often given credit for having the most advanced player development process. Through the use of levels in its minor league system, major league baseball develops young men who demonstrate talent but lack the experience and skills to currently succeed at the highest level of the sport. The Entrepreneurial League System (ELS) is a system that provides a comprehensive framework for developing small businesses from across five levels of development that metaphorically corresponds to the levels used in baseball—Rookie, A, AA, AAA, and the Majors.

Four dimensions define the characteristics (skills) of the entrepreneur to allow for an establishment of their ranking in the ELS. These dimensions are:

- *Technical skills.* Skill set of the entrepreneur necessary to complete key operations of the business enterprise
- *Managerial* skills. Skill set of the entrepreneur necessary to lead and supervise the business enterprise
- Entrepreneurial *skills.* Skill set to the entrepreneur to recognize market opportunities and develop creative strategies to capture those opportunities
- *Personal maturity.* Psychological and moral development characteristics of the entrepreneur that are related to business success

To facilitate the management of individual entrepreneurs through the levels, an assessment tool, the Entrepreneurial League System Assessment (ELSA) is designed to translate the essential concepts that are important in the development of entrepreneurship into an assessment framework, so that individuals can identify where they stand in the development of the needed skill set to create a successful small business. The ELSA uses the following action levels to define its responses:

0 Need for intensive action. Business cannot advance without addressing this item.
1 Need for action. The business must develop on this item prior to any successful launch.
2 Acceptable but opportunities for improvement exist. The business is ready on this item but could get better.
3 Optimal, no need for action. The item reflects a clear strength of the business.

Item Structure

Items were generated for each of the four core dimensions to be assessed by the ELSA. There items were generated by the developers of the ELS model informed by their experiences with business development and in collaboration with a number of small business entrepreneurs with whom they had worked. The initial version of the tool is described in Table 7.1 based on the names of the items created.

Next, action levels were developed for each item using the action ratings described above. Again, the process was informed by a combination of experience and input from entrepreneurs. Table 7.2 provides two example questions from the ELSA. Included in these item examples are the types of questions a diagnostician (see the following) might ask to tap into these dimensions. There is no requirement that these questions to the entrepreneur represent the only input into the ratings of the items.

Table 7.1 The Entrepreneurial League Levels by Degree of Skill

	Skills			
League	Technical	Managerial	Entrepreneurial	Personal Maturity
Majors	Outstanding	Outstanding	Outstanding	Outstanding
AAA	High	High	High	High
AA	High	Medium	Medium	Medium
A	High/Medium	Low	Low	Low
Rookie	Low/No	Low/No	Low/No	Low/No

From Lichtenstein and Lyons (2001).

Table 7.2 An Example Item to be Used Within the Entrepreneurial League System Assessment

Distribution Channels	
Where do you sell your product or provide your service? How do you get your product/ service to these distribution channels? Do you have established relationships with these channels? Are your existing channels sufficient to meet your business plan? How do your distribution channels compare with your competition's?	
0	Entrepreneur has yet to identify or establish distribution channels
1	Entrepreneur has identified potential distribution channels but has not yet established them
2	Entrepreneur has adequate distribution channels
3	Entrepreneur has exceptional distribution channels that further business interests

Recommended Assessment Process

For the purposes of the ELSA, the entrepreneur might be an individual or a team. The process is intended to describe the leadership of the business; however, that might be configured for a specific enterprise. The intent of the ELSA is to support the entrepreneur so that he or she can work with outside help to understand and reflect on his, her, or their enterprise in a manner that facilitates business growth. Consistent with that philosophy, it is recommended to be administered by an outside observer or neutral party, someone who is not working inside the business nor someone who is decided whether to supply venture capital.

Just like the CANS and the INTERMED, although the entrepreneur fully participates in the assessment process, the ELSA is not intended to be a self-report survey. A trained business diagnostician is required. One who has been a successful entrepreneur is optimal. That diagnostician must have access to detailed information about the entrepreneur and his, her, or their business (based on direct observation). Precisely how the diagnostician collects the necessary information will depend on circumstances such as the nature of the business, the parties involved in the assessment process, etc.

It is difficult to establish a priori exactly the amount and source(s) of knowledge needed by the diagnostician in order to complete the ELSA. Thus, the diagnostician's judgment and discretion in deciding how and where to obtain information to complete the assessment are encouraged. For this reason diagnosticians should be knowledgeable about the target business enterprise and trained in the use of the ELSA. The concept of information integration is particularly important with this approach, as the business diagnosticians integrate information for potentially dramatically different sources depending on the nature of the business.

The ELSA is designed to be performed in collaboration with the entrepreneur and his, her, or their team, in a setting that encourages mutual respect and a learning organizational culture (Senge, 2006) on the part of both the entrepreneur and the diagnostician. The assessment is not assumed to be a one-way process. In fact, the assessment process itself it intended to support a transformational process with the entrepreneur and is intended to serve as the first step in the transformational process of the ELS.

Psychometric Characteristics of the ELSA

Of course, if the ELSA is to be used to study change over time, then it is necessary to subject it to traditional psychometric analyses to determine whether scoring by dimensions is justifiable and that the dimension scores are sensitive to change. The technical skills component contains only one item; therefore, item analyses are limited to intercorrelations with the other dimensions. Inter-item correlational analyses are presented for three subscales of the tool, Management Skills (Table 7.3), Entrepreneurial Skills (Table 7.4), and Personal Maturity (Table 7.5).

Application of Cronbach's alpha to the items of each of these scales indicates a high level of internal consistency reliability. Management skills was 0.81; Entrepreneurial Skills was 0.83; and Personal Maturity was 0.80. All three of these values for alpha suggest that combining the items into scales is justifiable based on the statistical relationship among the items within each scale. Table 7.6 displays the intercorrelations among the four dimension scores of the ELSA. The range of these correlations is from 0.43 (Technical and Entrepreneurial Skills) and 0.68 (Entrepreneurial Skills and Personal Maturity. Thus, the highest variance shared between two dimension scores is 46%. This finding, in combination with the alphas, suggests that the ELSA measures four distinct constructs, each with sufficient consistency.

Table 7.3 Item to Total Correlation and Item–Item Correlations for the Management Subscale

Item	Subscale Total	Management	Financial	Resource	Administration
Management	0.65	0.26			
Financial	0.64	0.26			
Human resource	0.66	0.55	0.52		
Administration	0.60	0.40	0.42	0.38	
Problem-solving	0.67	0.51	0.45	0.53	0.38

Table 7.4 Item Analysis of the Entrepreneurial Skills Subscale on the ELSA

Item	Entrepreneurial Skills Total	Identifying New Markets	Generating Innovative Solutions	Capturing Market Opportunities
Identifying new markets	0.84			
Generating innovative solutions	0.88	0.70		
Capturing market opportunities	0.85	0.64	0.71	
Adaptation skills	0.63	0.34	0.40	0.42

Table 7.5 Item Analysis of Personal Maturity Subscale of the ELSA

Item	Personal Maturity Total Score	Accountability	Creativity	Openness to Change	Emotional Coping
Accountability	0.68				
Creativity	0.70	0.43			
Openness to change	0.72	0.35	0.43		
Emotional coping	0.70	0.41	0.45	0.39	
Self-awareness	0.80	0.54	0.43	0.49	0.57

Table 7.6 Intercorrelations Among the Four Subscales of the ELSA

	Technical Skills	Managerial Skills	Entrepreneurial Skills
Managerial skills	0.52		
Entrepreneurial skills	0.43	0.59	
Personal maturity	0.45	0.64	0.68

Thus, despite its design differences from a psychometric tool, scale scores can be derived that achieve standards consistent with classical test theory.

Impact Analysis

The ELSA is well suited to evaluate in terms of its impact. The nature of the ELS approach is to provide businesses with an understanding of their current status in terms of business development and specific direction for that development. Specifically, the goal is to help entrepreneurs to develop their individual business skills so that they can, in turn, successfully develop their businesses. Although nuanced by all sorts of potential complexities, the evaluation of business development is reasonably straightforward. The business should grow and make money if it is to be defined as a successful business. The following are two analyses of the impact of the ELS using the ELSA.

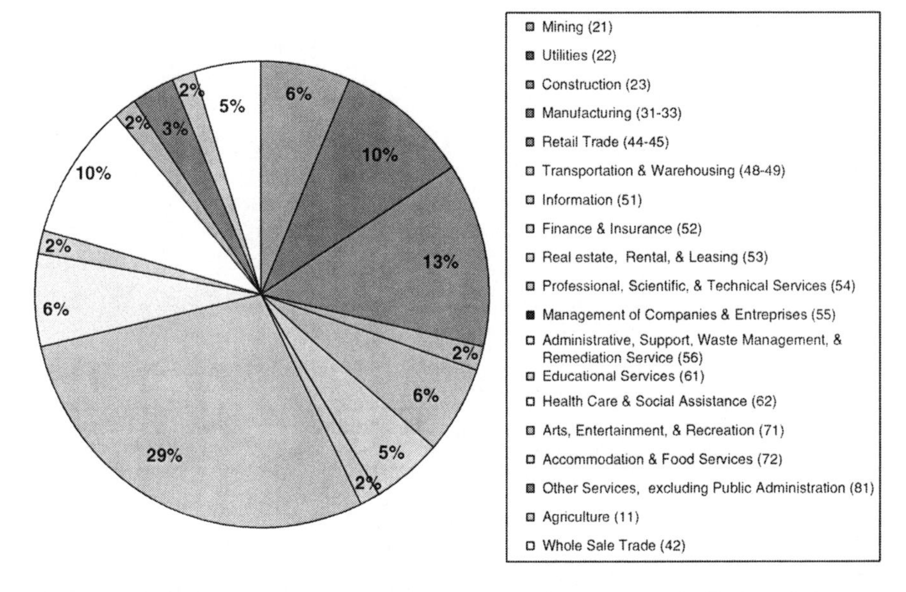

Fig. 7.1 NAICS (North American Industry Classification System) code distribution of advantage valley ELS clients.

ELS was implemented on November 1, 2004 with 24 entrepreneurs in the Advantage Valley in West Virginia. The present impact analysis ran through December 31, 2007. During the first 38 months, 112 clients participated (participation in the ELS is ramped up over time) and 66 (or 59%) remained active. Forty-five clients (40%) have exited the system; one (1%) graduated. Sixteen (14.3%) were placed in the stands. Of the 29 who exited the system, four were asked to leave because of unresponsive behavior,[1] three firms closed and six left for health or personal reasons. These movements in and out of the system are not unusual, and reflect the dynamic nature of business activity and entrepreneurship. Figure 7.1 presents the distribution of these businesses by type of enterprise.

The race of the entrepreneurs served by the ELS was consistent with the demographics of the population in which the businesses were located, although the vast majority were Caucasian (93%). About two-thirds of the entrepreneurs were men. Nine teams were developed to serve the participating businesses.

Table 7.7 provides the total sales revenues by ELS level. Note that the total sales average for the AA was 1.6 times that of the A, while the median sales average was 6.5 times. Additionally, the total sales average of the A was six times that of the Rookies, whereas the median sales average was 10.7 times. Clearly, ranking in the ELS model is related to business success from a sales volume perspective.

[1] Given the investment being made by the program sponsors, after a reasonable period during which every attempt was made to involve the entrepreneur in coaching, clients were dropped for non-participation.

Table 7.7 Total Sales Revenue Generated by ELS Clients Over a Six- (6) to Thirty-Eight- (38) Month Period as of 12/31/07

	All Skill Levels	Double A	Single A	Rookie
Number of clients	73	5	47	21
Total sales revenue	$55,445,274	$7,401,985	$44,705,844	$3,337,445
Percent of total sales	100%	13%	81%	6%
Average	$759,524	$1,480,397	$951,188	$158,926
Median	$206,092	$1,780,267	$273,604	$25,645
Maximum	$18,324,396	$2,366,705	$18,324,396	$1,647,567
Minimum	$100	$448,000	$2,072	$100

Table 7.8 Distribution of ELS clients in the pipeline by number of entrepreneurs in each skill level across stages of business development

Life cycle Skill Level	Stage 0Preventure	Stage 1Existence	Stage 2Early growth	Stage 3Expansion	Stage 4Maturity	Stage 5Decline
AAA(0)						
AA(5)			1	3	1	
A(53)	2	12	27	5	5	2
Rookie(8)	2	6				

To clarify the implications of the numbers in Table 7.7 it is useful to refer to another aspect of the ELS, referred to as the Pipeline of Entrepreneurs and Enterprises (Lichtenstein & Lyons, 2006). The concept of a "pipeline" of entrepreneurs and enterprises allows the segmentation of the marketplace of businesses by level of development. The pipeline contains two major variables: (1) skill level of the entrepreneur, and (2) stages in the development of the business (i.e., life cycle). These two variables can be combined to provide a new grid by which to view the community's business assets. Using this grid, the ELS clients can be sorted into the different segments of the marketplace. Table 7.8 reflects the distribution of ELS clients in this pipeline.

The average actual sales growth during the participation of these businesses in ELS was astronomical, at a more than 1.2 million percent increase. This was due to the fact that a number of companies were brand-new, with few if any sales, making for any growth being a large percentage of growth. The median growth was more than 100% for all business, with the larger median growth for Rookies at 123% followed by a robust 109% median growth from A level businesses. In terms of the impact of the investment in the system for each dollar spent on the ELS approach, it was $33 in revenue over the 38 months of the program.

The second impact analysis comes from an ELS implementation in central Louisiana. For this analysis, 1 year's worth of information—from June 1, 2006 to June 30th, 2007—was used. During this year, 51 clients were referred, and 41 were active at the end of the year. Six businesses were unresponsive and two failed. Three-fourths of the entrepreneurs were men and 85% were Caucasian.

Table 7.9 presents the growth during the year by level of ELS for the 20 clients who reported at least two quarters of sales information. Twenty-four companies participated at least two quarters of the year, but four did not report their sales for these analyses.

Table 7.9 Performance Measures For ELS as a Whole: One- (First) Year Quarterly Numbers

Performance Measures	As of 6/30/06	As of 6/30/07	Growth (loss), 12 Months	Growth (loss), %	Avg. Growth (loss)/Co.	Avg. Growth (loss), %/Co.
Number of clients	24	41	17	71%		
Number of clients reporting	20	41	21	105%		
Sales revenue	$3,679,726	$11,852,883	$8,173,157	222%	$199,345	5.4%
Employees	165	345	180	109%	4.4	2.7%
Revenue per employee	$22,301	$34,356	$12,055	54%	$294	1.3%
Sales outside region	$133,615	$1,945,366	$1,811,751	1,356%	$44,189	33%
Sales outside U.S.	$0	$2,515	$2,515	2,515%	$61	61%

Review of Table 7.9 reveals that the growth in real dollars averaged nearly $200,000 for each company, with an expansion of an average of 4.4 employees per enterprise. The growth in sales outside of the central Louisiana region is interesting from a business community perspective. Sales revenues from outside of the central Louisiana region increased by more than 1,300%. As such, the participating businesses were increasingly bringing new dollars into the region, which is a very important goal for an impoverished area.

Qualitative Analyses

The ELS also uses qualitative analyses to monitor the impact of its approach. These include interviews with coaches and participants.

One experienced coach described how he worked with an entrepreneur who doubted the coaching process:

> I mean, in other words I didn't tell him anything that he knew was wrong, but I asked him some questions that he was literally unable to answer and, given the context we'd just gone through of knowing how much money he would need to generate and how much he wanted to retire and everything, his inability to answer those questions made it clear to him that he wasn't going to be able to get from point A where he is now to point B where he wanted to be without being able to answer those questions. So, the whole coaching process was asking really good questions because I needed to know some of the answers in order for me to be helpful, but also I needed to have answers to questions—or he needed answers to these questions in order to know how to get from point A to point B. From a coaching approach, one of the key things to my success is *opening up his mind.* In Kutzhaova, Lyons, and Lichenstein (2008)

From the preceding discussion it should be apparent that the theory of communimetrics translates well outside of medical and behavioral health care. The use of a formal, action-oriented assessment strategy has been an essential component of a successful enterprise development strategy and provides both the structure for supporting transformation of business enterprises and a mechanism for evaluating the success of these enterprises. By elaborating the essential components of the business development strategy and operationalizing them into action-oriented items, the ELS becomes animated and understandable to the entrepreneur in a way that would not otherwise be possible.

Chapter 8
The Future of Measurement in Human Services Settings

This book outlines a theoretical framework with documented effectiveness in support of using structured assessment and the resulting numerical information to guide the evolution of transformational offering in human services enterprises. Not long ago this work might have been expected to have been met with skepticism, perhaps a yawn or a pat on the head. However, with the continued evolution of the information age, it is hard to imagine that human services enterprises will back away from the continued search for measurement strategies to support their work. In fact, there is every indication that the focus on measurement and performance in human services will be even more central to the operations of these fields in the future. With rapidly emerging information technologies that support the use of information in these settings, measurement in human services will continue to grow in importance.

An Integrative Model of Measurement

As discussed throughout this book, the various theories of measurement can be integrated into a single theory with a set of strategies. Communimetric and clinimetric approaches to measurement focus on the input side of the measurement process. Classical test theory and item response theory focus on the output side of the measurement process. In service delivery settings, it seems that communimetric and clinimetric theories have much to offer about the original design of a measurement approach. However, as soon as one wants to apply statistical analyses to information collected with these measures, considering of scaling characteristics for individual items (e.g., nominal, ordinal, interval) and scale characteristics for aggregate scores is necessary. Both of these processes are richly informed by the vast body of work on measurement theory and its applications.

It would not surprise me that some psychometricians might read this text and wish to argue that communimetrics is really already subsumed under existing psychometric theory. Certainly there could be an argument made for the complimentary nature of the approaches. They are not mutually exclusive, and as discussed in

J.S. Lyons, *Communimetrics: A Communication Theory of Measurement in Human Service Settings*,
DOI 10.1007/978-0-387-92822-7_8,

Chap. 4 and the three example chapters, if you want to use dimension scores from a communimetric tool, you need to honor the requirements set forward by psychometric measurement theories. However, you could develop and use a perfectly valid and reliable communimetric tool and never use dimension scores. Under those circumstances, you could completely ignore the test construction components of classical test and item response theories. You don't need to understand item difficulty or inter-item correlations. You do not have to care about factor structure or internal consistency reliability. You only have to worry about the scientific standards of all measurement—reliability and validity. And the specifics of these two core measurement constructs are different for measures designed to optimize communication.

Of course, only time and the input of others will resolve any dispute such as this one. Suffice it to say that I believe that shifting the priorities of the measurement enterprise to lead with communication as the most important objective results in a fundamental change in the value system used to create a good measure. The linking of the numbers on the rating scale to actions within the human service enterprise eliminates the arbitrary nature of measurement that haunts psychometrically developed tools. To me, these two distinctions are sufficient justification for a different theory of measurement. If anything, I might be prone to argue that psychometric analyses are subsumed under communimetrics when applied to field settings. The entire measurement process is a transaction that should first be understood within the context of its communication value.

Beyond inter-rater reliability, a communimetric measurement approach does not use the statistical performance of an item or items to guide the item development process. I have sat in on more than one consultation (and provided a few earlier in my career) in which the psychometrician argued for using an item's statistical performance to drive all decisions about item inclusion in a form. This strategy is a mistake when you would like people to embrace and actually use a measure. An egregious example of the downside of a purely psychometric approach comes from a measure of depression developed for elderly patients that we used in a study of an intervention for elderly patients who had broken their hips (Lyons, Strain, Hammer, Ackerman, & Fulop, 1989). There was one item on the measure that read, "Do you feel particularly helpless the way you are now?" When we used this measure in a study of the impact of a liaison intervention with these elderly fractured hip patients, it frequently generated an "affect storm." Typical responses included things like, "Well what the hell do you think . . . me lying here with my leg in a cast. . . ." Interviewers were frequently forced to distance themselves from the measure to maintain any credible relationship. They used statements such as, "I know sir. It's a stupid question, but it is part of a set of questions I'm supposed to ask. I really appreciate your help and I'm sorry about that question." I wonder whether there has been any research on the impact on reliability and validity of a classical test theory measure when the interviewer has to apologize for the insensitivity of a particular item? I don't know of any such research, but I'm confident the news would not be good.

Understanding Transformational Offerings

In health care and behavioral health care attention on outcomes has been growing for the past several decades (e.g., Lyons, Howard, O'Mahoney, & Lish, 1997). However, much of this work has still been embedded in a service delivery way of thinking about these human service enterprises. Other human services enterprises have even paid less attention to outcomes. Returning to Gilmore and Pine's (1997) conceptualization of offerings, it is clear that much of what is provided within human services enterprises are not really services, but rather transformation offerings. The goal of the enterprise is to help people change fundamental aspects of their lives, whether it is blood sugar levels, depression, housing stability, employment, or knowledge. As soon as you conceptualize human services enterprises as transformational offerings, it changes how you think about designing, managing, and evaluating them.

Further thinking about how to manage and maximize transformational offerings is an important goal of future work. As a foundation of that work, determining how best to measure and monitor transformational processes is a core innovation. While the study of change has a long and proud history in mental health (cf., Jacobson & Truax, 1991), it continues to require refinement and expansion to other areas in which people try to change their lives. Some outputs of transformational activities are straightforward: Weight loss can be measured in pound/kilograms or body fat. But to understand the actual process of transformation probably requires the measurement of intermediate processes (e.g., body image, knowledge of food, commitment to diet). It is unlikely that you can maximize the primary outcome of a weight loss program without also monitoring and managing some of the intermediate outcomes.

The ELSA is a good example of this challenge. The actual outcomes of a business can be reasonably straightforward in terms of revenue, employees, profit, etc. However, it is critical to understand the transformation of an entrepreneur from the time of the idea until the time the business has become successful according to standard financial outcome criteria.

Academic and Field Collaborations

Although there have been concerted efforts to bridge the gap, there is often a lack of effective collaboration between research and human services field applications. Often the academic field appears to take a transmission theory concept of communication with field applications. That is, academicians feel that they develop breakthroughs that should then be implemented by people working in applied fields. This mind set is reinforced by the nature of federal funding for research in field applications. No matter how creative a Request for Proposals might be in terms of seeking innovative collaborations between researchers and field settings, funding decisions continue to be made routinely by peer review panels populated primarily by researchers. This funding decision-making model merely reinforces the institutionalized way that many academicians think about field work. Phrases such as *knowledge transfer* and *dissemination of innovation* further reinforce our linear way of thinking about the relationship between academics and field applications.

It is seldom the case that researchers invent things that are then placed into practice, consistent with a transmission model of communication. Rather, moving to a constitutive conceptualization of this communication in which academic researchers and individuals working in field applications seek to develop a shared understanding of the work appears a more fruitful model for continued evolution of the field. I suggest that the concept is actually one of knowledge creation in which groups of people work together to create knowledge. Each person involved and exposed has an opportunity to influence the creation of the knowledge.

There are several ways in which communimetrics theory of measurement supports a reconceptualization of knowledge translation activities. First, the participation of all parties in the measurement process from development to use creates greater ownership of the results that come from measures. Second, the measures can be supported using reliable and valid measurement to inform management, and so the very process of implementing a measure assists individuals working in the field to value a research framework (e.g., TCOM). This process can serve to demystify the research enterprise. These measures from communimetric tools can be used to support valid research in field settings. The ability of academicians to engage in population-based research in field settings is enhanced substantially.

The great challenge of translating research into practice is that research must compete with experience and intuition to change the minds of people working in the field. By embedding itself into that experience, research activities have a substantially greater opportunity to become part of the experiences that influence people's knowledge (Lyons, 2009).

Mass Collaboration and Measurement Design, Development, and Use

Dramatic changes in information technology, demographics, and culture are changing the very nature of our economy (Tapscott & Williams, 2006). Old demarcations based on the proprietary nature of business and products are becoming obsolete in some markets. Opportunities for consumers to participate in the design of the products they buy are increasingly common. Mass collaborations are now possible. Wikipedia, MySpace, YouTube, the Human Genome Project, and so forth are revolutionizing how we think about community and the communal development of processes and products. These changes in how the information culture is changing business also have important implications for measurement.

Learning collaboratives have been advocated by many as vehicles of change (e.g., NCTSN, 2007). Convening people to work together for a common goal has been pursued using these strategies. Learning collaboratives are the model used within the Super User groups described in Chaps. 4 and 5.While learning collaboratives have significant advantages, they also suffer the limitation of requiring shared time. In the learning collaborative model, collaboratives must set aside the same time to meet in person, on the phone, or virtually in order to pursue the process. This aspect of the learning collaborative approach is a very limiting reality. Often, the spirit of collaboration exists but finding a common time to meet is very challenging and, at times, impossible. When schedules are forced, they can reduce the productivity of certain members. The larger the collaboration, the more difficult it becomes to manage the meetings. People can not all attend at the same time, and over time the process deteriorates because of inconsistent participation, which can easily be interpreted by fellow collaborators as a lack of commitment to the shared goals.

Mass collaborations use a different model (Tapscott & Williams, 2006). Metaphorically, a mass collaboration is like a very slow moving train on which people can jump on or off at any given time, regardless of the involvement of others in the collaboration at that moment in time. Individuals participating talk to each other, but the formal collaborative is not structured based on shared time, but on shared activities and experiences. Open source software is an example of mass collaborations. The three guiding principles are:

1. Nobody owns it.
2. Everybody uses it.
3. Any one can improve it.

In their breakthrough work, Tapscott and Williams (2006) argue that in the new digital economy, mass collaborations even among competing enterprises can be very good business. By reducing costs of infrastructure through sharing, businesses are poised to be more profitable in the long run. Human services enterprises are ideal markets for mass collaboration. The vast majority of these enterprises receive their funding directly or indirectly from government entities. There are three universal truths to this business environment:

1. There are many people in need.
2. Nobody has enough money to meet all of the need.
3. It is exceedingly difficult to get more money.

This creates a market with a great deal of unmet need. In the rare circumstance in which there is an expansion, it is quickly absorbed. In this business environment, effective efforts to reduce the costs of the infrastructure are an additional strategy to reach unmet need. Mass collaboration around assessment strategies that create information that can be used to better manage the transformational offerings in human services enterprises is a winning business strategy.

Despite the inherent logic to applying mass collaboration to the human services environment, there are many barriers to successful collaboration. These barriers can be categorized as threefold: ego, time and effort, and trust. In my experience, ego is the single biggest obstacle to effective mass collaboration. There are a variety of important reasons for this challenge. First, often people want credit for their work.

They need to feel that it is theirs—they own it. Agencies and programs often develop their own assessments, not because they will do it better than someone else, but because it will be their assessment. Unfortunately, these assessments are often poorly designed from a measurement perspective (e.g., too many open-ended questions or the inclusion of double-barreled questions) or even a forms management perspective (e.g., poor information flow), which further demoralize direct service staff on the value of standardized measurement.

If an academic is involved, one relatively straightforward route to tenure is to develop a measure and publish findings from it. The problem is acute in psychology with the classic example of Ogles, Lambert, and Masters' (1996) exhaustive review that identified more than 1,400 outcome measures in the published literature. Consistent with the culture, both of these authors then proceeded to develop their own measures—the Ohio Scales and the Outcome Questionnaire. Of course, the same applies to me. I recognize that I have based my own career on the development of measures. Thus, it is in my best interest for the measures I developed to flourish. Any success often will be at the expense of a different measurement option. This tension is not an easy one to resolve. It is certainly the case that academic innovation drives some aspects of system transformation. You certainly do not want to calcify the system in a way that thwarts this type of innovation. On the other hand, a plethora of options sometimes ends up paralyzing efforts to create a common language and approach.

Many academics also sell their assessment wares on the open market. Consequently, a conflict of interest between the intellectual value of measurement innovation and the financial benefit to the academic is possible. If you have a financial interest in the success of your measure, that changes the nature of the scientific enterprise for the involved parties. This potential conflict is a primary reason I first became interested in open source assessment strategies, which ultimately lead to mass collaboration. The core ethical consideration is that most research is funded in some manner by taxpayers. In my case, much of my research has been funded by state agencies responsible for serving high-need populations (e.g., mental health, child welfare). Personally profiting from the investments of these agencies seems immoral.

Until we reach a consensus in the field of measurement processes, it is likely that the value of new measurement development often will override efforts at mass collaboration. It is almost guaranteed that consensus on measurement will not come from the academic community. The famous meeting of psychotherapy outcome researchers at Vanderbilt is a good case example (Lyons, Howard, O'Mahoney, & Lish, 1997). At this meeting all of the leading experts were convened to try to reach a consensus on how to measure outcomes of psychotherapy. Each, of course, had developed his or her own measurement approach. For obvious reasons consensus on a specific measure was impossible. They could agree on what constructs should be measured—and that is feasible progress.

It is also unlikely that the mass collaboration will be directed from Washington, DC or any central government. Federal efforts at mandating standard assessment and measurement have experienced some successes, but have generally fallen short for all the reasons it is difficult to have a top-down process involving collaboration. The most likely approach will be a combination of a grassroots collaboration to build a growing consensus among those actually doing the work, followed by jurisdictional mandates to get those on board for those who for reasons of ego, time and effort, or trust failed to join the grassroots movement.

The second challenge to mass collaboration is time and effort. It can be difficult and time consuming to keep up with what others are doing and stay sufficiently current to be able to identify opportunities to join a mass collaboration. Technology innovations make this simpler today in some ways, but the sheer volume of the available information causes a new barrier of a similar type. It takes time and effort to collaborate.

The final challenge to mass collaboration is trust. If you talk to most high school students they have a great deal of trust in Wikipedia. Some use it as the primary source for many of their required papers. If you talk to most high school teachers they often express some distrust of this same collaboration. You have to be careful; the information is not always completely accurate. Trust is the foundation of communication. It is also the foundation of collaboration.

There are a number of reasons why we struggle with trust. Some challenges may result from our own personalities and personal experiences. Some people grow up trusting; others grow up cynical, distrustful, and even paranoid. The second challenge to trust comes from the marketplace. Competition, even in human services enterprises, exists among agencies that provide similar, related, or overlapping programs or interventions. This competition can undercut trust if competitors feel that they are losing an advantage by sharing. The third challenge is related to the time and effort barrier. Trust is a relational construct. It takes time and effort to build trust. You are much more likely to trust someone you know than someone you do not know. Building trust requires networking, time, and effort.

Trust is also an issue in mass collaboration from the developer's perspective. If you put your work out there in a mass collaboration, hopefully it will be used, but it may be misused. Fear of misuse can be a barrier to mass collaboration. No ethical measurement developer would want his or her tool misused. It is harder to manage the intellectual integrity of an approach when a mass collaboration strategy is employed.

Several of the currently developed communimetric tools have been created through processes of mass collaboration. The Praed Foundation holds the copyright on the Child and Adolescent Needs and Strengths and the Adult Needs and Strengths Assessment (ANSA) tools, but that is simply to ensure the intellectual integrity of the approach and keep the tools free to use (i.e., open domain). As described in Chap. 5, beginning with the initial design of the tool, many individuals had a great deal of input into the design. Over the years, different jurisdictions have contributed new items and strategies for use. In creating the Tennessee version, a psychiatrist in the development panel made the suggestion that sleep should be included. This question stimulated the creation of a sleep item that is now widely used. Similarly, having school representatives involved in the design phase resulted in Indiana developing an item to assess "bullying." This item has been integrated into a number of other versions.

The INTERMED uses a similar model for managing the tool with the INTERMED Foundation created to support its open use without cost. The INTERMED hasn't gone through as many versions as the CANS, but it is not yet as widely used. The creation of the version for the Case Management Society of America for use by case managers in the United States represents the first evolution of the tool in the fashion of a mass collaboration. A pediatric version of the tool is currently being developed with collaborators in Canada, the United States, and Europe.

If mass collaboration can become a foundation of measurement development for human service enterprises, some cultural change must occur. Tapscott and Williams (2006) outline a set of key strategies to use to try to make mass collaborations work.

> A new kind of business is emerging, one that opens the doors to the world, co-innovates with everyone, especially customers; shares resources that were previously closely guarded; harnesses the power of mass collaboration. . . . (p. 276).

These authors list four key principles:

1. *Being open*. Openness to new ideas and the opinions of others is a key to innovation and collaboration. It is easy to allow experience and the inertia that comes with it to lead us to complacency that we already have all the answers we need, and so we no longer ask questions. Often, the least experienced in an organization are the most open.
2. *Peering*. You can utilize the innovations of others by sharing those innovations. That's called peering. If you share a measurement process, any new strategies can be shared as well. An organization does not have to spend limited resources on development.
3. *Sharing*. "Smart firms today understand that sharing is more than playground etiquette" (Tapscott & Williams, 2006, p. 281). Sharing is a strategy to build trust, networks, collaborations, reduce costs, accelerate discoveries, and "lift the level of all boats."
4. *Acting globally*. Some jurisdictions become insular. They do not pay attention to anything that happens outside of their local context. This narrow vision is extremely limiting. Human services enterprises exist everywhere in the world. Postmodern technology facilitates the creation of global communications.

Mass collaboration is far less of an expert-based process than has currently been used in measurement development. Generally, a measure is developed by someone who is skilled in the techniques of measurement. Classical test theory and item response theory, which are both driven by the statistical performance of items within measures, require an expert driven process. Clinimetrics is more customer friendly in the sense that physicians should be partners in the development of measures. The measurement theory of communimetrics is even more consistent with the theory of mass collaboration. Customer and consumer should be involved in the design of each of the existing measures. They are active collaborators in the process. After all, the measure exists for their benefit. As such, they deserve credit for the measures as much as the expert who leads the process.

Because of the circumstances of the human services enterprises market, the value of mass collaboration in this sector is potentially enormous. If we can learn to work together to overcome the challenges of ego, time and effort, and trust, the value of these collaborations to the people we serve could be significant.

Increasing the Use of Measurement in Human Services Enterprises

As discussed throughout this book, there is a growing interest in and use of measurement strategies to inform the transformational offerings within the human services enterprise. However, these applications are relatively new and by no means close to universal. There remains much work to accomplish to prepare this sector for the optimal use of measurement in the management of the enterprise.

The Application of Information Technology

The dawning of the information age has seen the rapid development of information management capacities over the past 30 years. Just in my professional career we have witnessed incredible changes in the possibilities. The first document I ever word processed was my dissertation. In 1981, this was accomplished on a mainframe computer the size of a large room. I had to send each printing to a batch printer and wait in a large room for an output clerk to bin the printed copy. It generally took 15 to 30 minutes to receive an output. E-mail and the Internet were accessible only to a few scientists. Now, of course, my laptop is more powerful than that enormous machine and I can print in my office or send the document around the world electronically.

The implementation of applications from this technological innovation has been uneven generally, driven by a combination of available resources, interest, and perceived utility in the sector. I think it is fair to say that technological innovation has lagged somewhat behind in human services enterprises compared with most other business sectors. I believe the reason for this delay is threefold. First, as discussed, this sector does not have a lot of money. As such, human services enterprises do not generally have large budgets to spend on the development of technology. While vendors create technology for human services enterprise applications, the margin of profitability compared with other industries is likely to be far less than with other businesses.

Second, in this sector the value of technology might be perceived as lower. The priority of what limited resources are available is generally targeted on people. So, the ethos of the professions is more likely toward full employment than streamlining operations to reduce human capital costs. A major economic value of information technology is increasing productivity by reducing the time it took people to complete tasks that can be done easily electronically. That replacement inevitably results in either job loss or job restructuring.

Third, it has been my experience that people who are drawn to technology are a different group of people than those drawn to helping others. Sometimes people committed to careers in the service of others are not particularly interested in or skilled with information technology. Therefore, the field is populated with a somewhat larger prevalence of technophobic people, making innovation and implementation a bit more challenging. This problem is fading rapidly, however, with the reality that most college graduates have now grown up with technology. They were using computers when they were in preschool. I have not seen any formal studies on this topic, but it is probably safe to speculate that the number of people who are technophobic among the cohort of current leaders in the field who are 45 years and older is much higher than among the cohort of future leaders age 22 to 35.

Creating Innovative Applications of Measurement

A second necessary condition of expanding use is to develop a better fit between measurement applications and the management needs of human services enterprises. Historically, measurement has been tied to statistics and statistics have been tied to the general linear model. As discussed, the general linear model comes from a parametric model of statistics that requires assumptions to create computation convenience. With our current computing technology and access to populations, these assumptions are no longer requirements. With laptops nearly as powerful as the original supercomputers and databases routinely involving thousands or even tens of thousands of observations, parametric statistical approaches are not essential. Other approaches to the statistical manipulation of measures may be more desirable.

Rethinking the relationship of measurement to analysis is critical to opening up the potential for innovation applications. I presented two novel approaches in this book. First, the use of geomapping technology to map the relationship of actionable needs to available programs/interventions is a topographic approach that has obvious utility at the individual level, but also at the program and system levels for managing transformational offerings. Eventually, these systems can match by location and best outcomes for people with specific needs and/or strengths.

Particularly interesting applications of technology involve radically different analytical approaches that have been traditionally used to understand human services enterprises. Notable among these are geomapping approaches, which allow for a topographical analysis of an area in terms of matching people with available interventions. Recently a map was generated using a decision model from the CANS to identify the number of children and youth in child welfare who are indicated for a group home level of care by their home address along with a the physical location of the available group homes. The preponderance of group homes were located in different neighborhoods than the preponderance of youth who fit the CANS group home criteria, which suggested a gap in services. When the Director of IDCFS presented this map to Chicago aldermen, instead of reacting with the "not in my backyard" mentality to the concept of new group homes, the alderman with a higher number of youth but no group homes asked, "Why don't I have a group home in my district?" That thinking is a fundamental shift from the TCOM framework described earlier. "I have the people with needs. I want the ability to address their needs."

This particular application from which Figure 8.1 was developed is a platform that allows caseworkers to match the identified needs of children and youth with the nearest available provider and understand any special service that provider offers (e.g., evidence-based practices, day care, alternative languages). By closely linking the assessment to referral information, the value of the measurement is enhanced because it directly benefits the caseworker in completing his or her responsibilities.

Second, optimal data analysis (and related statistical approaches) is a nonparametric technique that identifies decision trees that map the characteristics of people to decisions made in a fashion that is completely impossible with general linear model techniques. As shown in Chap. 5, these models can be very revealing with regard to the relationship of the presentation of people to programs and the decisions made. The decision tree output of these approaches is far more intuitively obvious to people working in the field, making this a more accessible statistical analysis to study and improve decision validity.

Analytical innovations also would include generating reports and analyses that are useful to supervisors, managers, systems analysts, and leadership groups. In health care, there has been an evolution from report cards to dashboards to provide information that is intended to be helpful to systems. Report cards are static reports generated at fixed time points (e.g., quarterly, annually). Dashboards, on the other hand, are real-time reports that provide immediate status information on the functioning of a program/intervention and/or system. Creating useful dashboards is an

IDCFSSPD

CANS Recommended Services Report

DCFS ID W2166805 6227 S BISHOP ST FL 2
CHICAGO, IL 606362315

CANS

CANS Item	CANS Score	Service Type	Date of Assessment
4. Neglect	2		2008-09-17
10. Traumatic Grief/Separation	2		2008-09-17
14. Adjustment to Trauma	2	Individual Counseling/Therapy	2008-09-17
19. Family	2		2008-09-17
21. Educational	3		2008-09-17
22. Vocational	2		2008-09-17
23. Well-being	2		2008-09-17
25. Talents/Interests	2		2008-09-17
27. Community Life	2		2008-09-17
28. Relationship Permanence	2		2008-09-17
29. Family	2	Family Counseling/Therapy	2008-09-17
30. Living Situation	2	Family Counseling/Therapy	2008-09-17
33. Recreational	2	Recreational Activities	2008-09-17
34. Job Functioning	3		2008-09-17
35. Legal	2		2008-09-17
39. School Behavior	3		2008-09-17
40. School Achievement	2	Tutoring	2008-09-17
41. School Attendance	2		2008-09-17
50. Oppositional	2	Individual Counseling/Therapy Family Counseling/Therapy	2008-09-17
56. Anger Control	2	Individual Counseling/Therapy Anger Management/Conflict Resolution	2008-09-17
90. Educational Attainment	2		2008-09-17

W2168805 Page 1 of 109 09/24/2008 01:28:24 PM

Fig. 8.1 Example service recommendation report based on the Illinois Department of Children and Family Services version of the CANS

important priority as reliable and consistent measurement approaches increase in human service enterprises. Research on how information is used for managing transformational offerings is an important avenue of investigations. The best way to maximize use validity is to increase the usefulness of the information. Figure out what information provided in what time frames and which format to maximize utility is important to the evolution of this approach. How do you maximize the communication value of the information?

Creating Consumers of Information

Related to both aspects of innovation described in the preceding is how to create human capital skilled in the use of measurement outputs. Traditionally, measurement skills have been relegated to program evaluation or quality improvement specialists. Increasingly, all supervisors and managers must have skills in at least understanding the outputs of measurement process. If you can't manage what you don't measure, then you also can't manage if you don't understand what you are measuring or what it means when you do measure. Building the measurement and information intelligence of all employees in the human services enterprise is an important priority. Some expertise in program evaluation is now considered a core competency for receiving a doctorate in clinical psychology in the United States and Canada. This requirement is progress in the right direction. Similar core competencies in social work and public administration are equally important to the development of these professions.

Human services enterprises are businesses that seek to do good work by helping others. They often serve as a safety net for those of us who struggle at some point in our lives. Helping these individuals in their moment of need is the core principle of these enterprises. To better serve people in need, it is first important to know what they need. It is next important to be able to manage the enterprises with information about the degree to which these needs have been met. This is the core challenge of human services, and it is the mission of the communimetrics theory of measurement. By viewing assessment in these settings as a constitutive, "meaning-making" process between the individual or family in need and the people trying to help, communimetrics seeks to provide the strategy to allow this work to remain always about the people we serve.

References

Aarts, J., Ash, J., & Berg, M. (2007). Extending the understanding of computerized physician order entry: implications for professional collaboration, workflow and quality of care. *International Journal of Medical Informatics*, *76S*, S4–S13.

Achenbach, T. (1991). *Integrative guide to the 1991 CBCL/4 to 18, YSR, and TSR profiles*. Burlington, VT: University of Vermont, Department of Psychology.

Allen, M. J., & Yen, W. M. (2002). Introduction to Measurement Theory. Long Grove, IL: Waveland Press.

American Psychiatric Association (1980). *Diagnostic and statistical manual of psychiatric disorders* (3rd ed.). Washington, DC: American Psychiatric Association Press.

American Psychiatric Association (2004). *Diagnostic and statistical manual of mental disorder* (4th ed.). *Text Revision (DSM-IV TR)*. Washington, DC: American Psychiatric Association Press.

Anastasi, A. (1968). *Psychological testing* (3rd ed.). Toronto, ON, Canada: The Macmillan Company.

Anderson, J. A. (1996). *Communication theory: Epistemological foundations*. New York: Guildford Press.

Anderson, R. L., Lyons, J. S., Giles, D. M., Price, J. A., & Estle, G. (2003). Examining the reliability of the child and adolescent needs and strengths-mental health (CANS-MH) scale. *Journal of Child and Family Studies*, *12*, 1573–2843.

Apgar, V. (1966). The newborn (Apgar) scoring system. Reflections and advice. *Pediatric Clinics of North America 13*, 645–650.

Baggs, J. G., Ryan, S. A., Phelps, C. E., Richeson, J. F., & Johnson, J. E. (1992). The association between interdisciplinary collaboration and patient outcomes in an medical intensive care unit. *Heart Lung*, *21*, 18–24.

Bakeman, R., & Gottman, J. M. (1997). *Observing interaction* (2nd ed.). Cambridge, England, Cambridge University Press.

Bal, R., Mastboom, F., Spiers, H. P., & Rutten, H. (2007). The product and process of referral optimizing general practitioner-medical specialists' interaction trough information technology. *International Journal of Medical Informatics*, *76S*, S28–S34.

Behn, R. D. (2003). Why measure performance? Different purposes require different measures. *Public Administration Review*, *63*, 586–606.

Bell, V., Halligan, P. W., & Ellis, H. D. (2006). The cardiff anomalous perceptions scale (CAPS): A new validated measure of anomalous perceptual experience. *Schizophrenia Bulletin* 2006 *32(2)*, 366–377.

Beuscart-Zephir, M. -C., Pelayo, S., Anxeaux, F., Maxwell, D., & Suerlinger, S. (2007). Cognitive analysis of physician and nurses' cooperation in the medication ordering and administration process. *International Journal of Medical Informatics*, *76S*, S65–S77.

Bickman, L., Lambert, E. W., Andrade, A. R., & Penaloza, R. V. (2000). The Fort Bragg continuum of care for children and adolescents: mental health outcomes over 5 years. Journal of *Consulting and Clinical Psychology*, *68*, 710–716.

Blanton, H., & Jaccard, J. (2006). Arbitrary metrics in psychology. *American Psychologist*, *61*, 27–41.

Bloem, R. B., Beckley, D. J., van Hilten, B. J., & Roos, R. A. (1998). Clinimetrics of postural instability in Parkinson's disease. *Journal of Neurology, 245*, 669–673.

Boyle, D. K., & Kochinda, C. (2004). Enhancing collaborative communication of nurse and physician leadership in two intensive care units. *Journal of Nursing Administration, 34*, 60–70.

Brestan, E. V., & Eyberg, S. M. (1998), Effective psychosocial treatments of conduct-disordered children and adolescents: 29 years, 82 studies, and 5,272 kids. *Journal of Clinical Child Psychology, 27*, 180Y189

Butcher, J. N., Dahlstrom, W. G., Graham, J. R., Tellegen, A., & Kaemmer, B. (1989). *The Minnesota Multiphasic Personality Inventory-2 (MMPI-2): Manual for administration and scoring*. Minneapolis, MN: University of Minnesota Press.

Capaldi, E. J., & Proctor, R. W. (2000). Laudan's normative naturalism: A useful philosophy of science for psychology. *American Journal of Psychology, 115*, 430–454.

Carey, J. W. (1989). *Communication as culture: Essays on media and society*. Winchester MA: Unwin Hyman.

Chor, B (2008). Outcomes associated with following CANS recommendations for residential treatment.\Paper presented to the 5th annual CANS Conference, Nashville, TN, September

Ciechanowski, P. S., Katon, W. J., & Ruson, J. E. (2000). Depression and diabetes: impact of depressive symptoms on adherence, function and costs. *Archives of Internal Medicine, 160*, 3278–3285.

Cook, A., Spinazzola, J., Ford, J., Lanktree, C., Blaustein, M., Cloitre, M., et al. (2005). Complex trauma in children and adolescents. *Psychiatric Annals, 35*, 390–398.

Cook, T (2007). Measurement in children's services. Presented to the 16th annual System of Care conference at the Louis de la Parte Florida Mental Health Institute, March.

Craig, N., & MacIntyre, D. (2008). *The CANS with family support*. Paper presented at the 5th Annual CANS Conference, Nashville, TN.

Cronbach, L. J. (1951). Coefficient alpha and the internal structure of tests. *Psychometrika, 16(3)*, 297–334.

Curley, C., McEachern, J. E., & Speroff, T. (1998). A firm trial of interdisciplinary rounds on the inpatient medical wards. *Medical Care, 36*, AS4–AS12.

D'Agostino, Jr., R. B. (1998). Tutorial in biostatistics: propensity score methods for bias reduction in the comparison of a treatment to a non-randomized control group. *Statistics in Medicine, 17*, 2265–2281.

Dahlstrom, W. G., Brooks, J. D., & Peterson, C. D. (1990). The Beck depression inventory: Item order and the impact of response sets. *Journal of Personality Assessment, 55*, 225–233.

Deetz, S. A. (1994). Future of the discipline: The challenges, the research, and the social contribution. In S. A. Deetz (Ed.), *Communication Yearbook* 17 (pp. 565–600). Thousand Oaks, CA: Sage.

De Jonge, P., Huyse, F. J., Herzog, T., Lobo, A., Slaets, J. P., Lyons, J. S., et al. (2001). Risk factors for complex care in general medical inpatients: results from a European study. *Psychosomatics, 42*, 213–221.

De Jonge, P., Huyse, F. J., & Steifel, F. C. (2006). Case and care complexity in the medically ill. In F. J. Huyse & F. C. Steifel (Eds.), *Integrated care for the complex medically ill. The clinics of North America*. Philadelphia, PA: W.B. Saunders Company.

De Jonge, P., Ormel, J., & Slaets, J. P. J. (2004). Depressive symptoms in the elderly predict poor adjustment following somatic events. *American Journal of Geriatric Psychiatry, 12*, 57–64.

Dimatteo, M. R., Lepper, H. S., & Croghan, T. W. (2000). Depression is a risk factor for noncompliance with medical treatment. *Archives of Internal Medicine, 160*, 2101–2107.

Donsbach, W. (2006). The identify of communications research. *Journal of Communication, 56*, 437–448.

Doucette, A (2007). Measurement properties. Child and adolescent needs and strengths (CANS). *4th Annual CANS Conference*, Boston, October.

Dovey, S. M., Meyers, D. S., Phillips, R. L., Jr. (2002). A preliminary taxonomy of medical errors in family practice. *Quality & Safety in Health Care, 11*, 233–238.

Drucker, P. (1954). *The practice of management*. New York, NY: Harper Row.

Druss, B. (2006). Foreward. In F. J. Huyse & F. C. Steifel, (Eds.), *Integrated care for the complex medically ill. The Clinics of North America* (pp xiii–xiv). Philadelphia, PA: W.B. Saunders Company.

Duncan, T. E., Duncan, S. C., Strycker, L. A., Li, F., & Alpert, A. (1999). *An introduction to latent variable growth curve modeling: concepts, issues, and applications*. Mahwah, NJ: LEA.
Durr, M., Lyons, T. S., and Lichtenstein, G. A. (2000). Identifying the unique needs of urban entrepreneurs: African American skill set development. *Race & Society, 3*, 75–90.
Endicott, J., Spitzer, R. L., Fleiss, J. L., & Cohen, J. (1976). The global assessment scale. A procedure for measuring overall severity of psychiatric disturbance. *Archives of General Psychiatry, 33*, 766–771.
Epstein, M. H. (1998). Strength-based assessment: The behavioral and emotional rating scale. *Behavioral Healthcare Tomorrow, 7*, 46–48.
Elder, N. C., & Dovey, S. M. (2002). Classification of medical errors and preventable events in primary care: A synthesis of the literature. *The Journal of Family Practice, 51*, 927–932.
Epstein, R. M. (1995). Communication between primary care physicians and consultants. *Archives of Family Medicine, 4*, 403–409.
Eysenck, H. J. (1971). On the choice of personality tests for research and prediction. *Journal of Behavioural Science*, 1(3), 85–89.
Fava, G. A., & Belaise, C. (2005). A discussion of the role of clinimetrics and the misleading effects of psychometric theory. *Journal of Clinical Epidemiology, 58*, 753–756.
Feinstein, A. R. (1997). *Clinimetrics*. Yale University Press, New Haven.
Feinstein, A. R. (1999). Multi-item 'instruments' vs. Virginia Apgar's principles of clinimetrics. *Archives of Internal Medicine, 159*, 125–128.
Fenigstein, A., & Levine, M. P. (1984). Self-attention, concept activation, and the causal self. *Journal of Experimental Social Psychology, 20*, 231–245.
Friedland, L. A. (2001). Communication, community, and democracy: Toward a theory of communicatively integrated community. *Communication Research, 28*, 358–391.
Fogel, R. (1964). *Railroads and American economic growth. Essays in econometric history*. Baltimore: John Hopkins Press.
Fulop, G., Strain, J. J., Vita, G., Hammer, J., & Lyons, J. (1989). Diagnostic-related groups, psychiatric co-morbidities and prolonged length of stay. *Hospital & Community Psychiatry, 40*, 80–82.
Gandhi, T. K., Sittig, D. F., Franklin, M., Sussman, A. J., Fairchild, D. G., & Bates, D. W. (2000). Communication breakdown in the outpatient referral process. *Journal of General Internal Medicine, 15*, 626–631.
Gates, G. A., (2000). Clinimetrics of Meniere's disease. *Laryngoscope, 110*, 8–11.
Gilmore, J. H., & Pine B. J. (1997). Beyond goods and services. *Strategies & Leadership, 25(3)*, 10–17.
Hamilton, J. C., & Shuminsky, T. R. (1990). Self-awareness mediates the relationship between serial position and item reliability. *Journal of Personality and Social Psychology, 59*, 1301–1307.
Hancock, B. (2008). *Evaluating New Jersey's system of care*. Paper presented to the 5th Annual CANS Conference, Nashville, TN.
Harris, C. W. (Ed.). (1967). *Problems in measuring change*. Madison, Wisconsin: University of Wisconsin Press.
He, X. Z., Lyons, J. S., & Heinemann, A. W. (2004). Modeling crisis decision making for children in state custody. *General Hospital Psychiatry, 26*, 378–383.
Healy, K. (2005). *Social work theories in context*. Hampshire: Palgrave McMillan.
Hempel, C. (1950). Problems and changes in the empiricist criterion of meaning. *Revue Internationale de Philosophie 41*, 41–63.
Hodges, K., & Wotring, J. (2000). Client typology based on functioning across domains using the CAFAS: implications for service planning. *Journal of Behavioral Health Services & Research, 27*, 257–270.
Hoff, J. I., van Hilten, B. J., & Roos, R. A. (1999). A review of the assessment of dyskinesias. *Movement Disorders, 14*, 737–743.
Horn, S. (1983). Measuring severity of illness. Comparison across institutions. *American Journal of Public Health, 83*, 25–35.
House, J. S. (2002). Understanding social factors and inequality in health: 20th century progress and 21st century prospects. *Journal of Health and Social Behavior, 43*,125–142.
Howard, K. I., Kipta, M., Krause, M. S., & Orlinsky, D. E. (1986). The dose-effect relationship in psychotherapy. *American Psychologist, 41*, 159–163.

Huyse, F. J., Herzog, T., Malt, U., & Lobo, A. (1996). The European Consultation Liaison Workgroup. I. General Outline. *General Hospital Psychiatry, 18*, 44–55.

Huyse, F. J., Lyons, J. S., Stiefel, F. C., Slaets, J. P. J., De Jonge, P., Fink, P., et al. (1999). "INTERMED": A method to assess health service needs. I. Development and reliability. *General Hospital Psychiatry, 21*, 39–48.

Huyse, F. J., Lyons, J. S., Stiefel, F. C., Slaets, J., De Jonge, P., & Latour, C. (2001). Operationalizing the biopsychosocial model. The INTERMED. *Psychosomatics, 42*, 5–13.

Huyse, F. J., & Steifel, F. C. (Eds.). (2006). *Integrated care for the complex medically ill. The Clinics of North America.* Philadelphia, PA: W.B. Saunders Company.

Institute of Medicine (2001). *Crossing the quality chasm: A new health system for the 21st century. Committee on Quality of Health Care in America.* Washington, DC: National Academy Press.

Jacobson, N. S., & Truax, P. (1991). Clinical significance: A statistical approach to defining meaningful change in psychotherapy research. *Journal of Consulting and Clinical Psychology, 59*, 12–19.

Jaeschke, R., Singer, J., & Guyatt, G. H. (1990). A comparison of seven-point and visual analogue scales. Data from a randomized trial. *Controlled Clinical Trials, 11*, 43–51.

Kazdin, A. E. (2005). *Parent management training: Treatment for oppositional, aggressive, and antisocial behavior in children and adolescents.* New York, NY: Oxford University Press

Kijak, M., & Funtowicz, S. (1982). The syndrome of the survivor of extreme situations. *International Review of Psychoanalysis, 9*, 25–33.

Kitzinger J. (1994). The methodology of focus groups: the importance of interactions between research participants. *Sociology of Health and Illness, 16*, 103–121.

Knowles, E. S. (1988) Item context effects on personality scales: Measuring changes the measure. *Journal of Personality and Social Psychology, 55*, 312–320.

Krueger, R. A. and Casey, M. A. (2000). *Focus groups: A practical guide for applied research.* Thousand Oaks, CA: Sage Publications

Kuhn, T. (1962). *The Structure of Scientific Revolution.* Chicago, IL: University of Chicago Press.

Kutzhaova, N., Lyons, T. S., & Lichenstein, G. (2008). *Skills-based development of entrepreneurs and the role of personal and peer group coaching in enterprise development.* Working paper. Lawrence N. Field Center for Entrepreneurship, Baruch College, City University of New York.

Lambert, M. J., Ogles, B. M., & Masters, K. S. (2000). Choosing outcome assessment devices: An organizational and conceptual scheme. *Journal of Counseling and Development, 70*, 527–532.

Larson, E., Hamilton, H. E., Mitchell, K., & Eisenberg, J. (1998). Hospitalk: An exploratory study to asses what is said and what is heard between physicians and nurses. *Clinical Performance and Quality Health Care, 6*, 183–189.

Laudan, L. (1990). Normative naturalism. *Philosophy of Science, 57*, 44–59.

Leigh, H., Feinstein, A. R., & Reiser, M. F. (1980). The patient evaluation grid: a systematic approach to comprehensive care. *General Hospital Psychiatry, 2*, 3–9.

Lichtenstein, G. A., & Lyons, T. S. (2001). The entrepreneurial development system: Transforming business talent and community economies. *Economic Development Quarterly, 15(1)*, 3–20.

Lichtenstein, G., & Lyons, T. S. (2006). Managing the community's pipeline of entrepreneurs and enterprises: A new way of thinking about business assets. *Economic Development Quarterly, 20*, 377–386.

Lyles, A. (2002). Direct marketing of pharmaceuticals to consumers. *Annual Review of Public Health, 23*, 73–91.

Lyons, J. S. (2004). *Redressing the emperor: Improving our children's public mental health service system.* New York, NY: Praeger.

Lyons, J. S. (2009). Knowledge creation through Total Clinical Outcomes Management: A practice-based evidence solution to address some of the challenges of knowledge translation. JCACAP, *18*, 39–46.

Lyons, J. S., Cain, L. P, & Williamson, S. H. (2008). *Reflections on the Cliometrics Revolution. Conversations with Economic Historians.* New York, NY, Routledge.

Lyons, J. S., Colletta, J., Devens, M., & Finkel, S. I. (1995). The validity of the severity of psychiatric illness in a sample of inpatients are a psychogeriatric unit. *International Psychogeriatrics, 7*, 407–416.

Lyons, J. S., Griffin, G., Jenuwine, M., Shasha, M., & Quintenz, S. (2003). The mental health juvenile justice initiative. Clinical and forensic outcomes for a state-wide program. *Psychiatric Services, 54*, 1629–1634.

Lyons, JS, Howard, KI, O'Mahoney, MT, Lish, J (1997). *The measurement and management of clinical outcomes in mental health*. John Wiley & Sons, New York.

Lyons, J. S., Kisiel, C. L., Dulcan, M., Cohen, R., & Chesler, P. (1997). Crisis assessment and psychiatric hospitalization of children and adolescents in state custody. *Journal of Child and Family Studies, 6*, 311–320.

Lyons, J. S., Larson, D. B., Burns, B. J., Cope, N., Wright, S., & Hammer, J. S. (1988). Psychiatric co-morbidities in head and spinal cord injuries. Effects on acute hospital care. *General Hospital Psychiatry, 10*, 292–297.

Lyons, J. S., Mintzer, L. L., Kisiel, C. L., & Shallcross, H. (1998). Understanding the mental health needs of children and adolescents in residential treatment. *Professional Psychology: Research and Practice, 29*, 582–587.

Lyons, J. S., O'Mahoney, M. T., Larson, D. B. (1991). The attending psychiatrist as a predictor of length of stay. *Hospital and Community Psychiatry, 42*, 1064–1066.

Lyons, J. S., Rawal, P., Yeh, I., Leon, S., & Tracy, P. (2001). Use of measurement audit in outcomes management. *Journal of Behavioral Health Services & Research, 29*, 75–80.

Lyons, J. S., Rosen, A. J., & Dysken, M. (1985). Behavioral effects of drugs in depressed inpatients. *Journal of Consulting and Clinical Psychology, 53*, 17–24.

Lyons, J. S., Strain, J. J., Hammer, J. S., Ackerman, A. D., & Fulop, G. (1989). Reliability, validity, and temporal stability of the geriatric depression scale in hospitalized elderly. *International Journal of Psychiatry in Medicine, 19*, 205–211.

Lyons, J. S., Uziel-Miller, N. D., Reyes, F., & Sokol, P. T. (2000). The strengths of children and adolescents in residential settings: Prevalence and associations with psychopathology and discharge placement. *Journal of the Academy of Child and Adolescent Psychiatry 39*, 176–181.

Lyons JS & Weiner, DA (Editors) (2009). Strategies in Behavioral Healthcare: Total Clinical Outcomes Management. New York: Civic Research Institute.

Lyons, JS, Woltman, H, Martinovich, Z, Hancock, (2009). The role of residential treatment in a system of care. An outcome perspective. *Residential Treatment for Children and Youth* (forthcoming).

Makary, M. A., Sexton, J. B., Freischlag, J. A., Holzmueller, C. G., Millman, E. A., Rowen, L., & Pronovost, P. J. (2006). Operating room teamwork among physicians and nurses: teamwork in the eye of the beholder. *Journal of the American College of Surgeons, 202*, 746–752.

Manicas, P. T. (2006). *A realist philosophy of social science: explanation and understanding*. Cambridge, UK: Cambridge University Press.

Marshall, M. N. (1998). How well do general practitioners and hospital consultants work together? A qualitative study of cooperation and conflict within the medical profession. *British Journal of General Practice, 48*, 1379–1382.

Marx, R. G., Bombardier, C., Hogg-Johnson, S., & Wright, J. G. (1999). Clinimetric and psychometric strategies for development of a health measurement scale. *Journal of Clinical Epidemiology, 52*, 105–111.

Marx, R. G., Bombardier, C., Hogg-Johneon, S., & Wright, J. G. (2000). Clinimetric and psychometric strategies for development of a health measurement scale. *Journal of Clinical Epidemiology, 52*, 105–111.

McHorney, C. A., Ware, J. E., & Raczek, A. E. (1993). The MOST 36-item short-form health survey (SF-36) II. Psychometric and clinical tests of validity in measuring physical and mental health constructs. *Medical Care, 31*, 247–363.

McNally, R. J. (2004). Conceptual problems with the DSM-IV criteria for posttraumatic stress disorder. In G. M. Rosen (Ed.), *Posttraumatic stress disorder: Issues and controversies* (pp. 1–14). Chichester, UK: Wiley.

Meyers, P. C., & Budowski, M. (1995). Effects of organizing voluntary help on social support, stress and health of elderly people. *Clinical Society Review*, *13*, 106–119.

Mulder, CL, van der Graaff PCA, de Jonge P, de Groot AA, Lyons JS. (2000). Predicting admissions in emergency psychiatry. *European Psychiatry*, *15*, 313S.

Mulder, CL, Koopmans, GT, Lyons, JS (2005). The admission process untangled. Determinants of indicated versus actual level of care in psychiatric emergency services. Psychiatric Services *56*, 452–457.

Myers, C. S. (1940). *Shell shock in France 1914–1918*. Cambridge, UK: Cambridge University Press.

National Child Traumatic Stress Network. (2007). *Learning collaborative information packet*. Washington, DC: Substance Abuse and Mental Health Service Administration.

Newton, J., Hutchinson, A., Hayes, V., McColl, E., Mackee, I., & Holland, C. (1994). Do clinicians tell each other enough? An analysis of referral communications in two specialists. *Family Practice*, *11*, 15–20.

Nunally, J. (1976). *Psychometric theory* (2nd ed.). New York, NY: McGraw-Hill.

O'Brien, J., & Schneider, A. (2007). *CANS and service planning*. Workshop presented to the 4th Annual CANS Conference, Boston, MA.

Ogles, B. M., Lambert, M. J., & Masters, K. S. (1996). *Assessing outcome in clinical practice* (p 212). Needham Heights, MA: Allyn & Bacon, Inc.

Olson, E. E., Eoyard, G. H., Beckard, R., & Vaill, P. (2001). *Facilitating organization change: lessons from complexity science*. New York, NY: Pfeiffer.

Page, H. (1885). Injuries of the spine and spinal cord without apparent mechanical lesion. London: J&A Churchill.

Pavin, C. (1999) The third way: Scientific realism and communication theory. *Communication Theory*, *9(2)*, 162–188.

Pearce, W. B. (1989). *Communication and the human condition*. Carbondale: Southern Illinois University Press.

Peters, JD (1989). John Locke, the individual, and the origin of communication. *Quarterly Journal of Speech*, *75*, 387–399.

Phipps, L. M., Thomas, N. J. (2007). The use of daily goals sheet to improve communication in the paediatric intensive care unit. *Intensive and Critical Care Nursing*, *23*, 264–271.

Popper, K. R. (1959). *The logical of scientific discover*. New York, NY: Basic Books.

Pronovost, P., Berenholtz, S., Dorman, T., Lipsett, P. A., Simmonds, T., & Haraden, C. (2003). Improving communication in the ICU using daily goals. *Journal of Critical Care*, *18*, 71–75.

Rasch, G. (1960/1980). *Probabilistic models for some intelligence and attainment tests*. (Copenhagen, Danish Institute for Educational Research), expanded edition (1980) with foreword and afterword by B.D. Wright. Chicago, IL: The University of Chicago Press.

Rawal, P. H., Anderson, T. R., Romansky, J. R., & Lyons, J. S. (2008). Using decision support to address racial disparities in mental health service utilization. *Residential Treatment for Children and Youth*, *25*, 73–84.

Rawal, P., Lyons, J. S., MacIntyre, J., & Hunter, J. C. (2003). Regional variations and clinical indicators of antipsychotic use in residential treatment: A four state comparison. *Journal of Behavioral Health Services and Research 31*, 178–188.

Rosen, L. D., & Weil, M. M. (1996). Easing the transition from paper to computer-based systems. In T. Trabin (Ed.), *The computerization of behavioral healthcare. How to enhance clinical practice, management, and communications* (pp. 87–107). San Fransisco, CA, Josey-Bass.

Rosenbaum, P. R., & Rubin, D. B. (1983). *The central role of propensity scores in observational studies for causal effects. Biometrika*, *70*, 41–55.

Rothenbuhler, E. W. (1998). *Ritual communication: From everyday conversation to medical ceremony*. Thousand Oaks, CA: Sage.

Rowe, R. E., Garcia, J., Macfarlane, A. J., & Davidson, L. L. (2001). Does poor communication contribute to stillbirths and infant deaths? A review. Journal of Public Health Medicine, *23*, 23–34.

Safran, C., Porter, D., Slack, W., & Bleich, H. C. (1987). Diagnosis related groups. A critical assessment of the provision for comorbidity. Medical Care, *25*, 1011–1014.

San Martin-Rodriguez, L., Beaulieu, M.-D., D'Amour, D. (2005). The determinants of successful collaboration: a review of theoretical and empirical studies. Journal of Interprofessional Care, 19(Suppl), 132–147.

Schmidt, I., Claesson, C. B., Westerholm, B., Nilsson, L. G., & Svarstad, B. L. (1998). *Journal of the American Geriatrics Society*, *46*, 46–57.

Schwartz, S. P. (Ed.). (1977). *Naming, necessity, and natural kinds*. Ithaca, NY: Cornell University Press.

Senge, P. (2006). *The fifth discipline: The art and practice of the learning organization*. New York, NY: Doubleday.

Shaw, P. (2002). *Changing conversations in organizations. A complexity approach to change*. New York, NY, Routledge.

Sheahan, J (2008). *Valley's economic health hinges on small business success*. Retrieved November 8, from http://www.Themorningcall.com.

Shepherd, GJ (1993). Building a discipline of communication. *Journal of Communication*, *43*, 83–91.

Shrout, P. E. and Fleiss, J. L. (1979). Intraclass correlations: Uses in assessing rater reliability. *Psychological Bulletin*, *86(2)*, 420–428.

Sidlow, R., Katz-Sidlow, R. J. (2006). Using a computerized sign-out system to improve physician-nurse communication. *Journal on Quality and Patient Safety*, *32*, 32–36.

Slade, M, Phelan, M, Thornicroft, G (1998) A comparison of needs assessment by staff and by an epidemiologically representative sample of patients with psychosis. Psychological Medicine, *28*, 543–550.

Smedly, B. D., Stith, A., & Nelson, A. R. (2003). *Unequal treatment: confronting racial and ethnic disparities in health care*. Washington, DC: The National Academies Press.

Smith, G. R., Rost, K., & Kashner, T. M. (1995). A trial of the effect of a standardized psychiatric consultation on health outcomes and costs in somatizing patients. *Archives of General Psychiatry*, *52*, 238–243.

Snowden, J. A., Leon, S. C., Bryant, F. B., & Lyons, J. S. (2007). Evaluating psychiatric hospital admission decisions for children in foster care: an optimal classification tree analysis. *Journal of Clinical Child and Adolescent Psychology*, *36*, 8–18.

Streiner, DL (2003). Clinimetrics and psychometrics: an unnecessary distinction. Journal of Clinical *Epidemiology*, *56*, 1142–1145.

Stiefel, F. C., De Jonge, P., Huyse, F. J., Gues, P., Slaets, J. P. J., Lyons, J. S., et al. (1999). "INTERMED": A method to assess health service needs. II Results on its validity and clinical use. *General Hospital Psychiatry*, *21*, 49–56.

Stiefel, F. C., De Jonge, P., Huyse, F. J., Slaets, J. P. J., Guex, P., Lyons, J. S., et al. (1999). INTERMED—An assessment and classification system for case complexity. *Spine*, *24*, 378–385.

Stiefel, F. C., Huyse, F. J., Sollner, W., Slaets, J. P. J., Lyons, J. S., Latour, C. H. M., et al. (2006). Operationalizing integrated care on a clinical level: the INTERMED project. In F. J. Huyse & F. C. Stiefel (Eds.), Integrated care for the complex medically ill. *Medical Clinics of North America*, *90(4)*, 713–758.

Stone, M., Salonen, D., Lax, M., Payne, U., Lapp, V., & Inman, R. (2001). Clinical and imaging correlates of response to treatment with infliximab in patients with anklylosing spondylitis. *Journal of Rheumatology*, *28*, 1605–1614.

Strain, J. J., Lyons, J. S., Hammer, J. S., Fahs, M., Lebovits, A., Paddison, P. A., et al. (1991). Cost offset effects of a psychiatric liaison intervention. *American Journal of Psychiatry*, *148*, 1044–1049.

Stroul, B. A. (1993). Systems of Care for Children and Adolescents with Severe Emotional Disturbances: What Are the Results? CASSP Technical Assistance Center. Washington, DC: Center for Child Health and Mental Health Policy Center. Georgetown University Child Development Center.

Stroul, B. A., & Freidman, R. M. (1986). *A system of care for severely emotionally disturbed children and youth*. Washington, DC: Georgetown University Child Development Center.

Tapscott, D., & Williams, A. D. (2006). *Wikinomics. How mass collaboration changes everything*. New York, NY: Portfolio.

Tellegen, A., Ben-Porath, Y. S., McNulty, J. L., Arbisi, P. A., Graham, J. R., Kaemmer, B. (2003). The MMPI-2 restructured clinical scales: Development, validation, and interpretation. Minneapolis, MN: University of Minnesota Press.

Toulmin, S. (1970). Reasons and causes. In R. Borger & F. Cioffi (Eds.), *Explanation in the behavioral sciences* (pp. 1–26). Cambridge, UK, Cambridge University Press.

Trimble, M. R. (1985). Post-traumatic stress disorder: History of a concept. In C. R. Figley (Ed.), Trauma and its wake. The study and treatment of post-traumatic stress disorder. New York, NY: Brunner/Mazel Publishers.

Tyler, T., Rasinski, K. A., & Spodick, N. (1985). Influence of voice on satisfaction with leaders. Exploring the meaning of process control. *Journal of Personality and Social Psychology, 48*, 72–81.

U.S. Surgeon General (2001). *Report of the United States Surgeon General's Conference on Children's Mental Health. A national action agenda*. Washington, DC: Department of Health and Human Services.

VanDenBerg, J. & Grealish, E. M. (1998). *The wraparound process. Training manual*. Pittsburgh, PA: Author.

van der Kolk, B. (2005). Developmental trauma disorder. *Psychiatric Annals, 35*, 401–408.

van Os, J., Altamura, C., Bobes, J., Gerlach, J., Hellewell, J. S. E, Kasper, S., & Naber, D., Robert, P. (2004). Evaluation of the two-way communication checklist as a clinical intervention. *British Journal of Psychiatry, 184*, 79–83.

van Os, J., Altamura, A. C., Bobes, J., Owens, D. C., Gerlach, J., Hellewell, J. S. E., Kasper, S., Naber, D., Tarrier, N. & Robert, P. (2002). 2-COM: an instrument to facilitate patient-professional communication in routine clinical practice. *Acta Psychiatrica Scandinavica, 106*, 446–452.

Vickers, A. J. (2001). The use of percentage change from baseline in a controlled trial is statistically inefficient. A simulation study. *BMC Medical Research Methodology, 1*, 1–6.

Ware, J. E., & Sherbourne, C. D. (1992). The MOS 36-item short-form health survey (SF-36). I. Conceptual framework and item selection. *Medical Care, 30*, 473–483.

Weiner, D. A., Schneider, A., & Lyons, J. S. (2008). Evidence-based treatments for trauma among culturally diverse foster care youth. *Child and Youth Services Review* (in press).

WHO (1990). "Interim proposal for a WHO staging system for HIV infection and Disease.". Weekly Epidemiology Record, 65(29): 221–224

Wright, B. D. (1997). A history of social science measurement. *Educational Measurement: Issues and Practices, Winter*, 33–45.

Wright, B. D., & Stone, M. H. (1979). *Best test design*. Chicago, IL: MESA Press.

Wulsin, L. R., Sollner, W., & Pincus, H. A. (2006). Models of integrated care. In Wulsin, L. R., Vaillant, G. E., & Wells, V. E. A systematic review of the mortality of depression. *Psychosomatic Medicine, 61*, 6–17.

Yohanna, D, Christopher, NJ, Lyons, JS, Miller, SI, Slomowitz, M, Bultemaa, JK (1998). Characteristics of short-stay admissions to a psychiatric inpatient service. *Behavioral Health Service and Research, 25*, 337–346.

Zigmond, A. S., & Snaith, R. P. (1983). The hospital anxiety and depression scale. *Acta Psychiatrica Scandinavica, 67*, 361–370.

Zyzanski, S. J., & Perloff, E. (1999). Clinimetrics and psychometrics work hand in hand. *Archives of Internal Medicine, 159*, 1816–1817.

Appendix
Child and Adolescent Needs and Strengths (CANS)

Comprehensive Assessment For

Illinois Department of Children and Family Services Manual

A large number of individuals have collaborated in the development of the CANS-Comprehensive. Along with the CANS versions for developmental disabilities, juvenile justice, and child welfare, this information integration tool is designed to support individual case planning and the planning and evaluation of service systems. The trauma items were developed in collaboration Cassandra Kisiel, Ph.D., Glenn Saxe, M.D., Margaret Blaustein, Ph.D, Heide Ellis, Ph.D. with the SAMHSA-funded National Child Traumatic Stress Network. The CANS-Comprehensive is an open domain tool for use in service delivery systems that address the mental health of children, adolescents, and their families. The copyright is held by the Buddin Praed Foundation to ensure that it remains free to use. For more information about alternative versions of the CANS to use please contact Melanie Lyons of the Foundation. For more information on the **CANS-Comprehensive IDCFS** assessment tool contact:

John S. Lyons, Ph.D.,
Mental Health Services and Policy Program
Northwestern University
710 N. Lakeshore Drive, Abbott 1206
Chicago, Illinois 60611
(312) 908-8972
Fax (312) 503-0425
JSL329@northwestern.edu

Dana Weiner, Ph.D.
Mental Health Services and Policy Program
Northwestern University
710 N. Lakeshore Drive, Abbott 1206
Chicago, Illinois 60611
Dsaw80@northwestern.edu

Cassandra Kisiel, Ph.D.
National Center for Child Traumatic Stress-UCLA
11150 West Olympic Boulevard, Suite 770
Los Angeles, CA 90064
(310) 235-2633 x223
Fax (310) 235-2612

Coding Definitions & Guidelines

Trauma Experiences

These ratings are made based on lifetime exposure of trauma

For **Trauma Experiences,** the following categories and action levels are used:

0 indicates a dimension where there is no evidence of any trauma of this type.
1 indicates a dimension where a single even trauma occurred or suspicion exists of trauma experiences.
2 indicates a dimension on which the child has experienced multiple traumas.
3 indicates a dimension describes repeated and severe trauma with medical and physical consequences.

1. SEXUAL ABUSE

This rating describes child's experience of sexual abuse or the impact of the abuse on child's functioning.

0 There is no evidence that child has experienced sexual abuse.
1 Child has experienced single incident sexual abuse with no penetration.
2 Child has experienced multiple incidents of sexual abuse without penetration or a single incident of penetration.
3 Child has experienced severe, chronic sexual abuse that could include penetration or associated physical injury.

2. PHYSICAL ABUSE

This rating describes the degree of severity of the child physical abuse.

0 There is no evidence that child has experienced physical abuse.
1 There is a suspicion that child has experienced physical abuse but no confirming evidence. Spanking without physical harm or intention to commit harm also qualifies.
2 Child has experienced a moderate level of physical abuse and/or repeated forms of physical punishment (e.g., hitting, punching).
3 Child has experienced severe and repeated physical abuse with intent to do harm and that causes sufficient physical harm to necessitate hospital treatment.

3. EMOTIONAL ABUSE

This rating describes the degree of severity of emotional abuse, including verbal and nonverbal forms.

0 **There is no evidence that child has experienced emotional abuse.**
1 **Child has experienced mild emotional abuse. For instance, child may experience some insults or is occasionally referred to in a derogatory manner by caregivers.**
2 **Child has experienced moderate degree of emotional abuse. For instance, child may be consistently denied emotional attention from caregivers, insulted or humiliated on an ongoing basis, or intentionally isolated from others.**
3 **Child has experienced significant emotional abuse over an extended period of time (at least one year). For instance, child is completely ignored by caregivers, or threatened/terrorized by others.**

4. NEGLECT

This rating describes the degree of severity of neglect.

0 **There is no evidence that child has experienced neglect.**
1 **Child has experienced minor or occasional neglect. Child may have been left at home alone with no adult supervision or there may be occasional failure to provide adequate supervision of child.**
2 **Child has experienced a moderate level of neglect. This may include occasional unintended failure to provide adequate food, shelter, or clothing with corrective action.**
3 **Child has experienced a severe level of neglect including prolonged absences by adults, without minimal supervision, and failure to provide basic necessities of life on a regular basis.**

5. MEDICAL TRAUMA

This rating describes the degree of severity of medical trauma.

0 **There is no evidence that child has experienced any medical trauma.**
1 **Child has experienced mild medical trauma including minor surgery (e.g. stitches, bone setting).**
2 **Child has experienced moderate medical trauma including major surgery or injuries requiring hospitalization.**
3 **Child has experienced life threatening medical trauma.**

6. WITNESS TO FAMILY VIOLENCE

This rating describes the degree of severity of exposure to family violence.

0 **There is no evidence that child has witnessed family violence.**
1 **Child has witnessed one episode of family violence.**
2 **Child has witnessed repeated episodes of family violence but no significant injuries (i.e. requiring emergency medical attention) have been witnessed.**

3 Child has witnessed repeated and severe episode of family violence or has had to intervene in episodes of family violence. Significant injuries have occurred and have been witnessed by the child as a direct result of the violence.

7. COMMUNITY VIOLENCE

This rating describes the degree of severity of exposure to community violence.

0 There is no evidence that child has witnessed or experienced violence in the community.
1 Child has witnessed occasional fighting or other forms of violence in the community. Child has not been directly impacted by the community violence (e.g., violence not directed at self, family, or friends) and exposure has been limited.
2 Child has witnessed the significant injury of others in his/her community, or has had friends/family members injured as a result of violence or criminal activity in the community, or is the direct victim of violence/criminal activity that was not life threatening, or has witnessed/experienced chronic or ongoing community violence.
3 Child has witnessed or experienced the death of another person in his/her community as a result of violence, or is the direct victim of violence/criminal activity in the community that was life threatening, or has experienced chronic/ongoing impact as a result of community violence (e.g., family member injured and no longer able to work).

8. SCHOOL VIOLENCE

This rating describes the degree of severity of exposure to school violence.

0 There is no evidence that child has witnessed violence in the school setting.
1 Child has witnessed occasional fighting or other forms of violence in the school setting. Child has not been directly impacted by the violence (e.g., violence not directed at self or close friends) and exposure has been limited.
2 Child has witnessed the significant injury of others in his/her school setting, or has had friends injured as a result of violence or criminal activity in the school setting, or has directly experienced violence in he school setting leading to minor injury, or has witnessed ongoing/chronic violence in the school setting.
3 Child has witnessed the death of another person in his/her school setting, or has had friends who were seriously injured as a result of violence or criminal activity in the school setting, or has directly experienced violence in the school setting leading to significant injury or lasting impact.

9. NATURAL OR MANMADE DISASTERS

This rating describes the degree of severity of exposure to either natural or man-made disasters.

0 There is no evidence that child has been exposed to natural or man-made disasters.
1 Child has been exposed to disasters second hand (i.e., on television, hearing others discuss disasters). This would include second hand exposure to natural disasters such as a fire or earthquake or man-made disaster, including car accident, plane crashes, or bombings.
2 Child has been directly exposed to a disaster or witnessed the impact of a disaster on a family or friend. For instance, a child may observe a caregiver who has been injured in a car accident or fire or watch his neighbor's house burn down.
3 Child has been directly exposed to a disaster that caused significant harm or death to a loved one or there is an ongoing impact or life disruption due to the disaster (e.g., house burns down, caregiver loses job).

10. TRAUMATIC GRIEF/SEPARATION

This rating describes the level of traumatic grief due to death or loss or separation from significant caregivers.

0 There is no evidence that child has experienced traumatic grief or separation from significant caregivers.
1 Child is experiencing some level of traumatic grief due to death or loss of a significant person or distress from caregiver separation in a manner that is appropriate given the recent nature of loss or separation.
2 Child is experiencing a moderate level of traumatic grief or difficulties with separation in a manner that impairs function in certain but not all areas. This could include withdrawal or isolation from others.
3 Child is experiencing significant traumatic grief or separation reactions. Child exhibits impaired functioning across several areas (e.g., interpersonal relationships, school) for a significant period of time following the loss or separation.

11. WAR AFFECTED

This rating describes the degree of severity of exposure to war, political violence, or torture. Violence or trauma related to Terrorism is not included here.

0 There is no evidence that child has been exposed to war, political violence, or torture.
1 Child did not live in war-affected region or refugee camp, but family was affected by war. Family members directly related to the child may have been exposed to war, political violence, or torture; family may have been forcibly displaced due to the war, or both. This does not include children who have lost one or both parents during the war.
2 Child has been affected by war or political violence. He or she may have witnessed others being injured in the war, may have family members who

were hurt or killed in the war, and may have lived in an area where bombings or fighting took place. Child may have lost one or both parents during the war or one or both parents may be so physically or psychologically disabled from war so that they are not able to provide adequate caretaking of child. Child may have spent extended amount of time in refugee camp.

3 Child has experienced the direct affects of war. Child may have feared for their own life during war due to bombings, shelling, very near to them. They may have been directly injured, tortured, or kidnapped. Some may have served as soldiers, guerrillas, or other combatants in their home countries.

12. TERRORISM AFFECTED

This rating describes the degree to which a child has been affected by terrorism. Terrorism is defined as "the calculated use of violence or the threat of violence to inculcate fear, intended to coerce or to intimidate governments or societies in the pursuit of goals that are generally political, religious, or ideological." Terrorism includes attacks by individuals acting in isolation (e.g. sniper attacks).

0 There is no evidence that child has been affected by terrorism or terrorist activities.

1 Child's community has experienced an act of terrorism, but the child was not directly impacted by the violence (e.g. child lives close enough to site of terrorism that they may have visited before or child recognized the location when seen on TV, but child's family and neighborhood infrastructure was not directly affected). Exposure has been limited to pictures on television.

2 Child has been affected by terrorism within his/her community, but did not directly witness the attack. Child may live near the area where attack occurred and be accustomed to visiting regularly in the past, infrastructure of child's daily life may be disrupted due to attack (e.g. utilities or school), and child may see signs of the attack in neighborhood (e.g. destroyed building). Child may know people who were injured in the attack.

3 Child has witnessed the death of another person in a terrorist attack, or has had friends or family members seriously injured as a result of terrorism, or has directly been injured by terrorism leading to significant injury or lasting impact.

13. WITNESS/VICTIM TO CRIMINAL ACTIVITY

This rating describes the degree of severity of exposure to criminal activity.

0 There is no evidence that child has been victimized or witnessed significant criminal activity.

1 Child is a witness of significant criminal activity.

2 Child is a direct victim of criminal activity or witnessed the victimization of a family or friend.

3 Child is a victim of criminal activity that was life threatening or caused significant physical harm or child witnessed the death of a loved one.

Traumatic Stress Symptoms

These ratings describe a range of reactions that children and adolescents may exhibit to any of a variety of traumatic experiences from child abuse and neglect to community violence to disasters.

For **Trauma Stress Symptoms,** the following categories and action levels are used:

0 indicates a dimension where there is no evidence of any needs.
1 indicates a dimension that requires monitoring, watchful waiting, or preventive activities.
2 indicates a dimension that requires action to ensure that this identified need or risk behavior is addressed.
3 indicates a dimension that requires immediate or intensive action.

14. ADJUSTMENT TO TRAUMA

This item covers the youth's reaction to any of a variety of traumatic experiences – such as emotional, physical, or sexual abuse, separation from family members, witnessing violence, or the victimization or murder of family members or close friends. This dimension covers both adjustment disorders and posttraumatic stress disorder from DSM-IV.

0 Child has not experienced any significant trauma or has adjusted well to traumatic experiences.
1 Child has some mild adjustment problems to trauma. Child may have an adjustment disorder or other reaction that might ease with the passage of time. Or, child may be recovering from a more extreme reaction to a traumatic experience.
2 Child has marked adjustment problems associated with traumatic experiences. Child may have nightmares or other notable symptoms of adjustment difficulties.
3 Child has post-traumatic stress difficulties as a result of traumatic experience. Symptoms may include intrusive thoughts, hyper-vigilance, constant anxiety, and other common symptoms of Post Traumatic Stress Disorder (PTSD).

15. REEXPERIENCING

These symptoms consist of difficulties with intrusive memories or reminders of traumatic events, including nightmares, flashbacks, intense reliving of the events, and repetitive play with themes of specific traumatic experiences. These symptoms are part of the DSM-IV criteria for PTSD.

0 This rating is given to a child with no evidence of intrusive symptoms.
1 This rating is given to a child with some problems with intrusions, including occasional nightmares about traumatic events.
2 This rating is given to a child with moderate difficulties with intrusive symptoms. This child may have more recurrent frightening dreams with or without recognizable content or recurrent distressing thoughts, images, perceptions, or memories of traumatic events. This child may exhibit trauma-specific reenactments through repetitive play with themes of trauma or intense physiological reactions at exposure to traumatic cues.
3 This rating is given to a child with severe intrusive symptoms. This child may exhibit trauma-specific reenactments that include sexually or physically traumatizing other children or sexual play with adults. This child may also exhibit persistent flashbacks, illusions, or hallucinations that make it difficult for the child to function.

16. AVOIDANCE

These symptoms include efforts to avoid stimuli associated with traumatic experiences. These symptoms are part of the DSM-IV criteria for PTSD.

0 This rating is given to a child with no evidence of avoidance symptoms.
1 This rating is given to a child who exhibits some problems with avoidance. This child may exhibit one primary avoidant symptom, including efforts to try and avoid thoughts, feelings, or conversations associated with the trauma.
2 This rating is given to a child with moderate symptoms of avoidance. In addition to avoiding thoughts or feelings associated with the trauma, the child may also avoid activities, places, or people that arouse recollections of the trauma.
3 This rating is given to a child who exhibits significant or multiple avoidant symptoms. This child may avoid thoughts and feelings as well as situations and people associated with the trauma and have an inability to recall important aspects of the trauma.

17. NUMBING

These symptoms include numbing responses that are part of the DSM-IV criteria for PTSD. These responses are not present before the trauma.

0 This rating is given to a child with no evidence of numbing responses.
1 This rating is given to a child who exhibits some problems with numbing. This child may have a restricted range of affect or an inability to express or experience certain emotions (e.g., anger or sadness).

2 This rating is given to a child with moderate difficulties with numbing responses. This child may have a blunted or flat emotional state or have difficulty experiencing intense emotions or feel consistently detached or estranged form others following the traumatic experience.
3 This rating is given to a child with significant numbing responses or multiple symptoms of numbing. This child may have a markedly diminished interest or participation in significant activities and a sense of a foreshortened future.

18. DISSOCIATION

Symptoms included in this dimension are daydreaming, spacing, or blanking out, forgetfulness, emotional numbing, fragmentation, detachment, and rapid changes in personality often associated with traumatic experiences. This dimension may be used to rate dissociative disorders (e.g., Dissociative Disorder NOS, Dissociative Identity Disorder) but can also exist when other diagnoses are primary (e.g., PTSD, depression).

0 This rating is given to a child with no evidence of dissociation.
1 This rating is given to a child with minor dissociative problems, including some emotional numbing, avoidance, or detachment, and some difficulty with forgetfulness, daydreaming, spacing, or blanking out.
2 This rating is given to a child with a moderate level of dissociation. This can include amnesia for traumatic experiences or inconsistent memory for trauma (e.g., remembers in one context but not another), more persistent or perplexing difficulties with forgetfulness (e.g., loses things easily, forgets basic information), frequent daydreaming or trance-like behavior, depersonalization and/or derealization. This rating would be used for someone who meets criteria for Dissociative Disorder Not Otherwise Specified or another diagnosis that is specified "with dissociative features."
3 This rating is given to a child with severe dissociative disturbance. This can include significant memory difficulties associated with trauma that also impede day to day functioning. Child is frequently forgetful or confused about things he/she should know about (e.g., no memory for activities or whereabouts of previous day or hours). Child shows rapid changes in personality or evidence of alternate personalities. Child who meets criteria for Dissociative Identity Disorder or a more severe level of Dissociative Disorder NOS would be rated here.

Child Strengths

For **Child's Strengths**, the following categories and action levels are used:

0 indicates a domain where strengths exist that can be used as a centerpiece for a strength-based plan

1 indicates a domain where strengths exist but require some strength building efforts in order for them to serve as a focus of a strength-based plan.
2 indicates a domain where strengths have been identified but that they require significant strength building efforts before they can be effectively utilized in as a focus of a strength-based plan.
3 indicates a domain in which efforts are needed in order to identify potential strengths for strength building efforts.

19. FAMILY

Family refers to all biological or adoptive relatives with whom the child or youth remains in contact along with other individuals in relationships with these relatives.

0 Significant family strengths. This level indicates a family with much love and mutual respect for each other. Family members are central in each other's lives. Child is fully included in family activities.
1 Moderate level of family strengths. This level indicates a loving family with generally good communication and ability to enjoy each other's company. There may be some problems between family members. Child is generally included.
2 Mild level of family strengths. Family is able to communicate and participate in each other's lives; however, family members may not be able to provide significant emotional or concrete support for each other. Child is often not included in family activities.
3 This level indicates a child with no known family strengths. Child is not included in normal family activities.

20. INTERPERSONAL

This rating refers to the interpersonal skills of the child or youth both with peers and adults.

0 Significant interpersonal strengths. Child is seen as well liked by others and has significant ability to form and maintain positive relationships with both peers and adults. Individual has multiple close friends and is friendly with others.
1 Moderate level of interpersonal strengths. Child has formed positive interpersonal relationships with peers and/or other non-caregivers. Child may have one friend, if that friendship is a healthy 'best friendship model.
2 Mild level of interpersonal strengths. Child has some social skills that facilitate positive relationships with peers and adults but may not have any current relationships, but has a history of making and maintaining healthy friendships with others.
3 This level indicates a child with no known interpersonal strengths. Child currently does not have any friends nor has he/she had any friends in the past. Child does not have positive relationships with adults.

21. EDUCATIONAL

This rating refers to the strengths of the school system and may or may not reflect any specific educational skills possessed by the child or youth.

0 This level indicates a child who is in school and is involved with an educational plan that appears to exceed expectations. School works exceptionally well with family and caregivers to create a special learning environment. A child in a mainstream educational system who does not require an individual plan would be rated here.
1 This level indicates a child who is in school and has a plan that appears to be effective. School works fairly well with family and caregivers to ensure appropriate educational development.
2 This level indicates a child who is in school but has a plan that does not appear to be effective.
3 This level indicates a child who is either not in school or is in a school setting that does not further his/her education.

22. VOCATIONAL

Generally this rating is reserved for adolescents and is not applicable for children 12 years and under. Computer skills would be rated here.

0 This level indicates an adolescent with vocational skills who is currently working in a natural environment.
1 This level indicates an adolescent with pre-vocational and some vocational skills but limited work experience.
2 This level indicates an adolescent with some pre-vocational skills. This also may indicate a child or youth with a clear vocational preference.
3 This level indicates an adolescent with no known or identifiable vocational or pre-vocational skills and no expression of any future vocational preferences.

23. WELL-BEING

This rating should be based on the psychological strengths that the child or adolescent might have developed including both the ability to enjoy positive life experiences and manage negative life experiences. This should be rated independent of the child's current level of distress.

0 This level indicates a child with exceptional psychological strengths. Both coping and savoring skills are well developed.
1 This level indicates a child with good psychological strengths. The person has solid coping skills for managing distress or solid savoring skills for enjoying pleasurable events.
2 This level indicates a child with limited psychological strengths. For example, a person with very low self-esteem would be rated here.

3 **This level indicates a child with no known or identifiable psychological strengths. This may be due to intellectual impairment or serious psychiatric disorders.**

24. OPTIMISM

This rating should be based on the child or adolescent's sense of him/herself in his/her own future. This is intended to rate the child's positive future orientation.

0 **Child has a strong and stable optimistic outlook on his/her life. Child is future oriented.**
1 **Child is generally optimistic. Child is likely able to articulate some positive future vision.**
2 **Child has difficulties maintaining a positive view of him/herself and his/her life. Child may vary from overly optimistic to overly pessimistic.**
4 **Child has difficulties seeing any positives about him/herself or his/her life.**

25. TALENT/INTERESTS

This rating should be based broadly on any talent, creative, or artistic skill a child or adolescent may have including art, theatre, music, athletics, etc.

0 **This level indicates a child with significant creative/artistic strengths. A child/youth who receives a significant amount of personal benefit from activities surrounding a talent would be rated here.**
1 **This level indicates a child with a notable talent. For example, a youth who is involved in athletics or plays a musical instrument, etc. would be rated here.**
2 **This level indicates a child who has expressed interest in developing a specific talent or talents even if they have not developed that talent to date.**
3 **This level indicates a child with no known talents, interests, or hobbies.**

26. SPIRITUAL/RELIGIOUS

This rating should be based on the child or adolescent's and their family's involvement in spiritual or religious beliefs and activities.

0 **This level indicates a child with strong moral and spiritual strengths. Child may be very involved in a religious community or may have strongly held spiritual or religious beliefs that can sustain or comfort him/her in difficult times.**
1 **This level indicates a child with some moral and spiritual strengths. Child may be involved in a religious community.**
2 **This level indicates a child with few spiritual or religious strengths. Child may have little contact with religious institutions.**
3 **This level indicates a child with no known spiritual or religious involvement.**

27. COMMUNITY LIFE

This rating should be based on the child or adolescent's level of involvement in the cultural aspects of life in his/her community.

0 This level indicates a child with extensive and substantial, long-term ties with the community. For example, individual may be a member of a community group (e.g. Girl or Boy Scout etc.) for more than one year, may be widely accepted by neighbors, or involved in other community activities, informal networks, etc.
1 This level indicates a child with significant community ties although they may be relatively short term (e.g. past year).
2 This level indicates a child with limited ties and/or supports from the community.
3 This level indicates a child with no known ties or supports from the community.

28. RELATIONSHIP PERMANENCE

This rating refers to the stability of significant relationships in the child or youth's life. This likely includes family members but may also include other individuals.

0 This level indicates a child who has very stable relationships. Family members, friends, and community have been stable for most of his/her life and are likely to remain so in the foreseeable future. Child is involved with both parents.
1 This level indicates a child who has had stable relationships but there is some concern about instability in the near future (one year) due to transitions, illness, or age. A child who has a stable relationship with only one parent may be rated here.
2 This level indicates a child who has had at least one stable relationship over his/her lifetime but has experienced other instability through factors such as divorce, moving, removal from home, and death.
3 This level indicates a child who does not have any stability in relationships.

Life Domain Functioning

For **Life Functioning Domains**, the following categories and action levels are used:

0 indicates a life domain in which the child is excelling. This is an area of considerable strength
1 indicates a life domain in which the child is doing OK. This is an area of potential strength
2 indicates a life domain in which the child is having problems. Help is needed to improve functioning into an area of strength.
3 indicates a life domain in which the child is having significant problems. Intensive help is needed to improve functioning into an area of strength.

29. FAMILY

Family ideally should be defined by the child; however, in the absence of this knowledge consider biological relatives and their significant others with whom the child still has contact as the definition of family.

0 Child is doing well in relationships with family members.
1 Child is doing adequately in relationships with family members although some problems may exist. For example, some family members may have some problems in their relationships with child.
2 Child is having moderate problems with parents, siblings and/or other family members. Frequent arguing, difficulties in maintaining any positive relationship may be observed.
3 Child is having severe problems with parents, siblings, and/or other family members. This would include problems of domestic violence, constant arguing, etc.

30. LIVING SITUATION

This item refers to how the child is functioning in their current living arrangement which could be a relative, a temporary foster home, shelter, etc.

0 No evidence of problem with functioning in current living environment.
1 Mild problems with functioning in current living situation. Caregivers concerned about child's behavior in living situation.
2 Moderate to severe problems with functioning in current living situation. Child has difficulties maintaining his/her behavior in this setting creating significant problems for others in the residence.
3 Profound problems with functioning in current living situation. Child is at immediate risk of being removed from living situation due to his/her behaviors.

31. SOCIAL FUNCTIONING

This item refers to the child's social functioning from a developmental perspective.

0 Child is on a healthy social development pathway.
1 Child is having some minor problems with his/her social functioning.
2 Child is having some moderate problems with his/her social functioning.
3 Child is experiencing severe disruptions in his/her social functioning.

32. DEVELOPMENTAL/INTELLECTUAL

This rating describes the child's development as compared to standard developmental milestones such as talking, walking, toileting, cooperative play, etc.

0 No evidence of developmental problems or mental retardation.
1 Evidence of a mild developmental delay or low IQ (70–85)

2 Evidence of a pervasive developmental disorder including Autism, Tourette's, Down's Syndrome or other significant developmental delay or child's has mild mental retardation (50-69).
3 Severe developmental disorder or IQ below 50.

33. RECREATIONAL

This item is intended to reflect the child access to and use of leisure time activities.

0 Child has and enjoys positive recreation activities on an ongoing basis.
1 Child is doing adequately with recreational activities although some problems may exist.
2 Child is having moderate problems with recreational activities. Child may experience some problems with effective use of leisure time.
3 Child has no access to or interest in recreational activities. Child has significant difficulties making use of leisure time.

34. JOB FUNCTIONING

This item is intended to describe functioning in vocational settings. If a child or youth is not working, rate a "3."

0 Child is gainfully employed in a job and performing well.
1 Child is gainfully employed but may have some difficulties at work.
2 Child works intermittently for money (e.g. babysitting) or child has job history but is currently not working.
3 Child has no job history.
NA Not applicable based on child's age.

35. LEGAL

This item involves only the child's (not the families') involvement with the legal system.

0 Child has no known legal difficulties.
1 Child has a history of legal problems but currently is not involved with the legal system.
2 Child has some legal problems and is currently involved in the legal system.
3 Child has serious current or pending legal difficulties that place him/her at risk for a court ordered out of home placement

36. MEDICAL

This item refers to the child's health.

0 Child is healthy.
1 Child has some medical problems that require medical treatment.
2 Child has chronic illness that requires ongoing medical intervention.
3 Child has life threatening illness or medical condition.

37. PHYSICAL

This item describes any physical limitations the child may experience due to health or other factors.

0 Child has no physical limitations.
1 Child has some physical condition that places mild limitations on activities. Conditions such as impaired hearing or vision would be rated here. Rate here, treatable medical conditions that result in physical limitations (e.g. asthma).
2 Child has physical condition that notably impacts activities. Sensory disorders such as blindness, deafness, or significant motor difficulties would be rated here.
3 Child has severe physical limitations due to multiple physical conditions.

38. SEXUAL DEVELOPMENT

This rating describes issues around sexual development including developmentally inappropriate sexual behavior and problematic sexual behavior. Sexual orientation or gender identity issues could be rated here if they are leading to difficulties.

0 No evidence of any problems with sexual development.
1 Mild to moderate problems with sexual development. May include concerns about sexual identity or anxiety about the reactions of others.
2 Significant problems with sexual development. May include multiple older partners or high-risk sexual behavior.
3 Profound problems with sexual development. This level would include prostitution, very frequent risky sexual behavior, or sexual aggression.

39. SCHOOL BEHAVIOR

This item rates the behavior of the child or youth in school or school-like settings (e.g. Head Start, pre-school). A rating of 3 would indicate a child who is still having problems after special efforts have been made, i.e., problems in a special education class.

0 No evidence of behavior problems at school or day care. Child is behaving well.
1 Mild problems with school behavioral problems. May be related to either relationships with teachers or peers. A single detention might be rated here.
2 Child is having moderate behavioral difficulties at school. He/she is disruptive and may receive sanctions including suspensions or multiple detentions.

3 Child is having severe problems with behavior in school. He/she is frequently or severely disruptive. School placement may be in jeopardy due to behavior.
NA Not applicable for children five years and younger

40. SCHOOL ACHIEVEMENT

This item describes academic achievement and functioning.

0 Child is doing well in school.
1 Child is doing adequately in school, although some problem with achievement exists.
2 Child is having moderate problems with school achievement. He/she may be failing some subjects.
3 Child is having severe achievement problems. He/she may be failing most subjects or is more than one year behind same age peers in school achievement.
NA Not applicable for children five years and younger

41. SCHOOL ATTENDANCE

If school is not in session, rate the last 30 days when school was in session.

0 No evidence of attendance problems. Child attends regularly.
1 Child has some problems attending school, although he/she generally goes to school. He/she may miss up to one day per week on average. Or, he/she may have mad moderate to severe problems in the past six months but has been attending school regularly in the past month.
2 Child is having problems with school attendance. He/she is missing at least two days per week on average.
3 Child is generally truant or refusing to go to school.

Acculturation

For **Acculturation,** the following categories and action levels are used:

0 indicates a dimension where there is no evidence of any needs.
1 indicates a dimension that requires monitoring, watchful waiting, or preventive activities.
2 indicates a dimension that requires action to ensure that this identified need or risk behavior is addressed.
3 indicates a dimension that requires immediate or intensive action.

42. LANGUAGE

This item includes both spoken and sign language.

0 Child and family speak English well.
1 Child and family speak some English but potential communication problems exist due to limits on vocabulary or understanding of the nuances of the language.
2 Child and/or significant family members do not speak English. Translator or native language speaker is needed for successful intervention but qualified individual can be identified within natural supports.
3 Child and/or significant family members do not speak English. Translator or native language speaker is needed for successful intervention and no such individual is available from among natural supports.

43. IDENTITY

Cultural identify refers to the child's view of his/herself as belonging to a specific cultural group. This cultural group may be defined by a number of factors including race, religion, ethnicity, geography, or lifestyle.

0 Child has clear and consistent cultural identity and is connected to others who share his/her cultural identity.
1 Child is experiencing some confusion or concern regarding cultural identity.
2 Child has significant struggles with his/her own cultural identity. Child may have cultural identity but is not connected with others who share this culture.
3 Child has no cultural identity or is experiencing significant problems due to conflict regarding his/her cultural identity.

44. RITUAL

Cultural rituals are activities and traditions that are culturally including the celebration of culturally specific holidays such as kwanza, cinco de mayo, etc. Rituals also may include daily activities that are culturally specific (e.g. praying toward Mecca at specific times, eating a specific diet, access to media)

0 Child and family are consistently able to practice rituals consistent with their cultural identity
1 Child and family are generally able to practice rituals consistent with their cultural identity; however, they sometimes experience some obstacles to the performance of these rituals.
2 Child and family experience significant barriers and are sometimes prevented from practicing rituals consistent with their cultural identity.
3 Child and family are unable to practice rituals consistent with their cultural identity.

45. CULTURE STRESS

Culture stress refers to experiences and feelings of discomfort and/or distress arising from friction (real or perceived) between an individual's own cultural identify and the predominant culture in which he/she lives.

0 **No evidence of stress between individual's cultural identify and current living situation.**
1 **Some mild or occasional stress resulting from friction between the individual's cultural identify and his/her current living situation.**
2 **Individual is experiencing cultural stress that is causing problems of functioning in at least one life domain.**
3 **Individual is experiencing a high level of cultural stress that is making functioning in any life domain difficult under the present circumstances.**

Child Behavioral/emotional Needs

For **Behavioral/Emotional Needs,** the following categories and symbols are used:

0 indicates a dimension where there is no evidence of any needs.
1 indicates a dimension that requires monitoring, watchful waiting, or preventive activities.
2 indicates a dimension that requires action to ensure that this identified need or risk behavior is addressed.
3 indicates a dimension that requires immediate or intensive action.

46. PSYCHOSIS

This item is used to rate symptoms of psychiatric disorders with a known neurological base. DSM-IV disorders included on this dimension are Schizophrenia and Psychotic disorders (unipolar, bipolar, NOS). The common symptoms of these disorders include hallucinations, delusions, unusual thought processes, strange speech, and bizarre/idiosyncratic behavior.

0 **This rating indicates a child with no evidence of thought disturbances. Both thought processes and content are within normal range.**
1 **This rating indicates a child with evidence of mild disruption in thought processes or content. The child may be somewhat tangential in speech or evidence somewhat illogical thinking (age inappropriate). This also includes children with a history of hallucinations but none currently. The category would be used for children who are subthreshold for one of the DSM diagnoses listed above.**
2 **This rating indicates a child with evidence of moderate disturbance in thought processes or content. The child may be somewhat delusional or have brief or intermittent hallucinations. The child's speech may be at times quite tangential or illogical. This level would be used for children who meet the diagnostic criteria for one of the disorders listed above.**
3 **This rating indicates a child with severe psychotic disorder. The child frequently is experiencing symptoms of psychosis and frequently has no reality assessment. There is evidence of ongoing delusions or hallucinations**

or both. Command hallucinations would be coded here. This level is used for extreme cases of the diagnoses listed above.

47. ATTENTION DEFICIT/IMPULSE CONTROL

Symptoms of Attention Deficit and Hyperactivity Disorder and Impulse Control Disorder would be rated here. Inattention/distractibility not related to opposition would also be rated here.

0 This rating is used to indicate a child with no evidence of attention/hyperactivity problems.
1 This rating is used to indicate a child with evidence of mild problems with attention/hyperactivity or impulse control problems. Child may have some difficulties staying on task for an age appropriate time period.
2 This rating is used to indicate a child with moderate symptoms attention/ hyperactivity or impulse control problems. A child who meets DSM-IV diagnostic criteria for ADHD would be rated here.
3 This rating is used to indicate a child with severe impairment of attention or dangerous impulse control problems. Frequent impulsive behavior is observed or noted that carries considerable safety risk (e.g. running into the street, dangerous driving or bike riding). A child with profound symptoms of ADHD would be rated here.

48. DEPRESSION

Symptoms included in this dimension are irritable or depressed mood, social withdrawal, and anxious mood; sleep disturbances, weight/eating disturbances, and loss of motivation. This dimension can be used to rate symptoms of the following psychiatric disorders as specified in DSM-IV: Depression (unipolar, dysthymia, NOS), Bipolar.

0 This rating is given to a child with no emotional problems. No evidence of depression.
1 This rating is given to a child with mild emotional problems. Brief duration of depression, irritability, or impairment of peer, family, or academic functioning that does not lead to gross avoidance behavior.
2 This rating is given to a child with a moderate level of emotional disturbance. This could include major, depression, or school avoidance. Any diagnosis of depression would be coded here. This level is used to rate children who meet the criteria for an affective disorder listed above.
3 This rating is given to a child with a severe level of depression. This would include a child who stays at home or in bed all day due to depression or one whose emotional symptoms prevent any participation in school, friendship groups, or family life. Disabling forms of depressive diagnoses would be coded here. This level is used to indicate an extreme case of one of the disorders listed above.

49. ANXIETY

This item describes the child's level of fearfulness, worrying, or other characteristics of anxiety.

0 No evidence of any anxiety or fearfulness.
1 History or suspicion of anxiety problems or mild to moderate anxiety associated with a recent negative life event. This level is used to rate either a mild phobia or anxiety problem or a sub-threshold level of symptoms for the other listed disorders.
2 Clear evidence of anxiety associated with either anxious mood or significant fearfulness. Anxiety has interfered significantly in child's ability to function in at least one life domain.
3 Clear evidence of debilitating level of anxiety that makes it virtually impossible for the child to function in any life domain

50. OPPOSITIONAL BEHAVIOR (Compliance with authority)

This item is intended to capture how the child relates to authority. Oppositional behavior is different from conduct disorder in that the emphasis of the behavior is on non-compliance to authority rather than on seriously breaking social rules, norms, and laws.

0 This rating indicates that the child/adolescent is generally compliant.
1 This rating indicates that the child/adolescent has mild problems with compliance to some rules or adult instructions. Child may occasionally talk back to teacher, parent/caregiver may be letters or calls from school.
2 This rating indicates that the child/adolescent has moderate problems with compliance to rules or adult instructions. A child who meets the criteria for Oppositional Defiant Disorder in DSM-IV would be rated here.
3 This rating indicates that the child/adolescent has severe problems with compliance to rules or adult instructions. A child rated at this level would be a severe case of Oppositional Defiant Disorder. They would be virtually always noncompliant. Child repeatedly ignores authority.

51. CONDUCT

These symptoms include antisocial behaviors like shoplifting, lying, vandalism, and cruelty to animals, assault. This dimension would include the symptoms of Conduct Disorder as specified in DSM-IV.

0 This rating indicates a child with no evidence of behavior disorder.
1 This rating indicates a child with a mild level of conduct problems. The child may have some difficulties in school and home behavior. Problems are recognizable but not notably deviant for age, sex, and community. This might include occasional truancy, repeated severe lying, or petty theft from family.

2 **This rating indicates a child with a moderate level of conduct disorder. This could include episodes of planned aggressive or other anti-social behavior. A child rated at this level should meet the criteria for a diagnosis of Conduct Disorder.**

3 **This rating indicates a child with a severe Conduct Disorder. This could include frequent episodes of unprovoked, planned aggressive or other anti-social behavior.**

52. SUBSTANCE ABUSE

These symptoms include use of alcohol and illegal drugs, the misuse of prescription medications and the inhalation of any substance for recreational purposes. This rating is consistent with DSM-IV Substance-related Disorders.

0 **This rating is for a child who has no substance use difficulties at the present time. If the person is in recovery for greater than 1 year, they should be coded here, although this is unlikely for a child or adolescent.**

1 **This rating is for a child with mild substance use problems that might occasionally present problems of living for the person (intoxication, loss of money, reduced school performance, parental concern). This rating would be used for someone early in recovery (less than 1 year) who is currently abstinent for at least 30 days.**

2 **This rating is for a child with a moderate substance abuse problem that both requires treatment and interacts with and exacerbates the psychiatric illness. Substance abuse problems consistently interfere with the ability to function optimally but do not completely preclude functioning in an unstructured setting.**

3 **This rating is for a child with a severe substance dependence condition that presents a significant complication to the coordination of care (e.g. need for detoxification) of the individual. A substance-exposed infant who demonstrates symptoms of substance dependence would be rated here.**

53. ATTACHMENT DIFFICULTIES

This item should be rated within the context of the child's significant parental or caregiver relationships.

0 **No evidence of attachment problems. Caregiver-child relationship is characterized by mutual satisfaction of needs and child's development of a sense of security and trust. Caregiver appears able to respond to child cues in a consistent, appropriate manner, and child seeks age-appropriate contact with caregiver for both nurturing and safety needs.**

1 **Mild problems with attachment. There is some evidence of insecurity in the child-caregiver relationship. Caregiver may at times have difficulty accurately reading child bids for attention and nurturance; may be inconsistent in response;**

or may be occasionally intrusive. Child may have mild problems with separation (e.g., anxious/clingy behaviors in the absence of obvious cues of danger) or may avoid contact with caregiver in age-inappropriate way. Child may have minor difficulties with appropriate physical/emotional boundaries with others.

2 **Moderate problems with attachment. Attachment relationship is marked by sufficient difficulty as to require intervention. Caregiver may consistently misinterpret child cues, act in an overly intrusive way, or ignore/avoid child bids for attention/nurturance. Child may have ongoing difficulties with separation, may consistently avoid contact with caregivers, and may have ongoing difficulties with physical or emotional boundaries with others.**

3 **Severe problems with attachment. Child is unable to form attachment relationships with others (e.g., chronic dismissive/avoidant/detached behavior in care giving relationships) OR child presents with diffuse emotional/physical boundaries leading to indiscriminate attachment with others. Child is considered at ongoing risk due to the nature of his/her attachment behaviors. A child who meets the criteria for an Attachment Disorder in DSM-IV would be rated here. Child may have experienced significant early separation from or loss of caregiver, or have experienced chronic inadequate care from early caregivers, or child may have individual vulnerabilities (e.g., mental health, developmental disabilities) that interfere with the formation of positive attachment relationships.**

54. EATING DISTURBANCES

These symptoms include problems with eating including disturbances in body image, refusal to maintain normal body weight and recurrent episodes of binge eating. These ratings are consistent with DSM-IV Eating Disorders.

0 **This rating is for a child with no evidence of eating disturbances.**

1 **This rating is for a child with a mild level of eating disturbance. This could include some preoccupation with weight, calorie intake, or body size or type when of normal weight or below weight. This could also include some binge eating patterns.**

2 **This rating is for a child with a moderate level of eating disturbance. This could include a more intense preoccupation with weight gain or becoming fat when underweight, restrictive eating habits or excessive exercising in order to maintain below normal weight, and/or emaciated body appearance. This level could also include more notable binge eating episodes that are followed by compensatory behaviors in order to prevent weight gain (e.g., vomiting, use of laxatives, excessive exercising). This child may meet criteria for a DSM-IV Eating Disorder (Anorexia or Bulimia Nervosa).**

3 **This rating is for a child with a more severe form of eating disturbance. This could include significantly low weight where hospitalization is required or excessive binge-purge behaviors (at least once per day).**

55. AFFECT DYSREGULATION

These symptoms include difficulties modulating or expressing emotions, intense fear or helplessness, difficulties regulating sleep/wake cycle, and inability to fully engage in activities.

0 This rating is given to a child with no difficulties regulating emotional responses. Emotional responses are appropriate to the situation.
1 This rating is given to a child with some minor difficulties with affect regulation. This child could have some difficulty tolerating intense emotions and become somewhat jumpy or irritable, in response to emotionally charged stimuli or more watchful or hypervigilant in general. This child may have some difficulty sustaining involvement in activities for any length of time.
2 This rating is given to a child with moderate problems with affect regulation. This child may be unable to modulate emotional responses. This child may exhibit marked shifts in emotional responses (e.g., from sadness to irritability to anxiety) or have contained emotions with a tendency to lose control of emotions at various points (e.g., normally restricted affect punctuated by outbursts of anger or sadness). This child may also exhibit persistent anxiety, intense fear or helplessness, or lethargy/loss of motivation.
3 This rating is given to a child with severe problems with highly dysregulated affect. This child may have more rapid shifts in mood and an inability to modulate emotional responses (feeling out of control of their emotions). This child may also exhibit tightly contained emotions with intense outbursts under stress. Alternately, this child may be characterized by extreme lethargy, loss of motivation or drive, and no ability to concentrate or sustain engagement in activities (i.e., emotionally "shut down").
NA Not applicable due to child's age. See section for children 0–5 years old.

56. BEHAVIORAL REGRESSIONS

These ratings are used to describe shifts in previously adaptive functioning evidenced in regressions in behaviors or physiological functioning.

0 This rating is given to a child with no evidence of behavioral regression.
1 This rating is given to a child with some regressions in age-level of behavior (e.g., thumb sucking, whining when age inappropriate).
2 This rating is given to a child with moderate regressions in age-level of behavior including loss of ability to engage with peers, stopping play or exploration in environment that was previously evident, or occasional bedwetting.
3 This rating is given to a child with more significant regressions in behaviors in an earlier age as demonstrated by changes in speech or loss of bowel or bladder control.

57. SOMATIZATION

These symptoms include the presence of recurrent physical complaints without apparent physical cause or conversion-like phenomena (e.g., pseudoseizures).

0 This rating is for a child with no evidence of somatic symptoms.
1 This rating indicates a child with a mild level of somatic problems. This could include occasional headaches, stomach problems (nausea, vomiting), joint, limb, or chest pain without medical cause.
2 This rating indicates a child with a moderate level of somatic problems or the presence of conversion symptoms. This could include more persistent physical symptoms without a medical cause or the presence of several different physical symptoms (e.g., stomach problems, headaches, backaches). This child may meet criteria for a somatoform disorder. Additionally, the child could manifest any conversion symptoms here (e.g., pseudoseizures, paralysis).
3 This rating indicates a child with severe somatic symptoms causing significant disturbance in school or social functioning. This could include significant and varied symptomatic disturbance without medical cause.

58. ANGER CONTROL

This item captures the youth's ability to identify and manage their anger when frustrated.

0 This rating indicates a child with no evidence of any significant anger control problems.
1 This rating indicates a child with some problems with controlling anger. He/she may sometimes become verbally aggressive when frustrated. Peers and family members are aware of and may attempt to avoid stimulating angry outbursts.
2 This rating indicates a child with moderate anger control problems. His/her temper has gotten him/her in significant trouble with peers, family, and/or school. This level may be associated with some physical violence. Others are likely quite aware of anger potential.
3 This rating indicates a child with severe anger control problems. His/her temper is likely associated with frequent fighting that is often physical. Others likely fear him/her.
NA Not applicable due to child's age.

Child Risk Behaviors

For **Risk Behaviors,** the following categories and action levels are used:

0 indicates a dimension where there is no evidence of any needs.
1 indicates a dimension that requires monitoring, watchful waiting, or preventive activities.

2 indicates a dimension that requires action to ensure that this identified need or risk behavior is addressed.
3 indicates a dimension that requires immediate or intensive action.

59. SUICIDE RISK

This rating describes both suicidal and significant self-injurious behavior. A rating of 2 or 3 would indicate the need for a safety plan.

0 Child has no evidence or history of suicidal or self-injurious behaviors.
1 History of suicidal or self-injurious behaviors or significant ideation but no self-injurious behavior during the past 30 days.
2 Recent, (last 30 days) but not acute (today) suicidal ideation or gesture. Self-injurious in the past 30 days (including today) without suicidal ideation or intent.
3 Current suicidal ideation and intent in the past 24 h.

60. SELF-MUTILATION

This rating includes repetitive physically harmful behavior that generally serves a self-soothing functioning with the child.

0 No evidence of any forms of self-mutilation (e.g. cutting, burning, face slapping, head banging)
1 History of self-mutilation but none evident in the past 30 days.
2 Engaged in self mutilation that does not require medical attention.
3 Engaged in self mutilation that requires medical attention.

61. OTHER SELF HARM

This rating includes reckless and dangerous behaviors that while not intended to harm self or others, place the child or others at some jeopardy. Suicidal or self-mutilative behavior is NOT rated here.

0 No evidence of behaviors that place the child at risk of physical harm.
1 History of behavior other than suicide or self-mutilation that places child at risk of physical harm. This includes reckless and risk-taking behavior that may endanger the child.
2 Engaged in behavior other than suicide or self-mutilation that places him/her in danger of physical harm. This includes reckless behavior or intentional risk-taking behavior.
3 Engaged in behavior other than suicide or self-mutilation that places him/her at immediate risk of death. This includes reckless behavior or intentional risk-taking behavior.

62. DANGER TO OTHERS

This rating includes actual and threatened violence. Imagined violence, when extreme, may be rated here. A rating of 2 or 3 would indicate the need for a safety plan.

0 **Child has no evidence or history of aggressive behaviors or significant verbal aggression towards others (including people and animals).**
1 **History of aggressive behavior or verbal aggression towards others but no aggression during the past 30 days. History of fire setting (not in past year) would be rated here.**
2 **Occasional or moderate level of aggression towards others including aggression during the past 30 days or more recent verbal aggression.**
3 **Frequent or dangerous (significant harm) level of aggression to others. Child or youth is an immediate risk to others.**

63. SEXUAL AGGRESSION

Sexually abusive behavior includes both aggressive sexual behavior and sexual behavior in which the child or adolescent takes advantage of a younger or less powerful child through seduction, coercion, or force.

0 **No evidence of problems with sexual behavior in the past year.**
1 **Mild problems of sexually abusive behavior. For example, occasional inappropriate sexually aggressive/harassing language or behavior.**
2 **Moderate problems with sexually abusive behavior, For example, frequent inappropriate sexual behavior. Frequent disrobing would be rated here only if it was sexually provocative. Frequent inappropriate touching would be rated here.**
3 **Severe problems with sexually abusive behavior. This would include the rape or sexual abuse of another person involving sexual penetration.**

64. RUNAWAY

In general, to classify as a runaway or elopement, the child is gone overnight or very late into the night. Impulsive behavior that represents an immediate threat to personal safety would also be rated here.

0 **This rating is for a child with no history of running away and no ideation involving escaping from the present living situation.**
1 **This rating is for a child with no recent history or running away but who has expressed ideation about escaping present living situation or treatment. Child may have threatened running away on one or more occasions or have a history (lifetime) of running away but not in the past year.**
2 **This rating is for a child who has run away from home once or run away from one treatment setting within the past year. Also rated here is a child who has run away to home (parental or relative) in the past year.**

3 This rating is for a child who has (1) run away from home and/or treatment settings within the last 7 days or (2) run away from home and/or treatment setting twice or more overnight during the past 30 days. Destination is not a return to home of parent or relative.

65. DELINQUENCY

This rating includes both criminal behavior and status offenses that may result from child or youth failing to follow required behavioral standards (e.g. truancy). Sexual offenses should be included as criminal behavior.

0 Child shows no evidence or has no history of criminal or delinquent behavior.
1 History of criminal or delinquent behavior but none in the past 30 days. Status offenses in the past 30 days would be rated here.
2 Moderate level of criminal activity including a high likelihood of crimes committed in the past 30 days. Examples would include vandalism, shoplifting, etc.
3 Serious level of criminal or delinquent activity in the past 30 days. Examples would include car theft, residential burglary, gang involvement, etc.

66. JUDGMENT

This item describes the child's decision-making processes and awareness of consequences.

0 No evidence of problems with judgment or poor decision making that result in harm.
1 History of problems with judgment in which the child makes decisions that are in some way harmful. For example, a child who has a history of hanging out with other children who shoplift.
2 Problems with judgment in which the child makes decisions that are in some way harmful to his/her development and/or well-being.
3 Problems with judgment that place the child at risk of significant physical harm.

67. FIRE SETTING

This item refers to behavior involving the intentional setting of fires that might be dangerous to the child or others. This does not include the use of candles or incense or matches to smoke.

0 No evidence or history of fire setting behavior
1 History or fire-setting but not in past six months
2 Recent fire setting behavior (in past six months) but not of the type that has endangered the lives of others (e.g. playing with matches) OR repeated fire

setting behavior over a period of at least two years even if not in the past six months.

3 **Acute threat of fire setting. Set fire that endangered the lives of others (e.g. attempting to burn down a house).**

68. SOCIAL BEHAVIOR

This rating describes obnoxious social behaviors that a child engages in to intentionally force adults to sanction him/her. This item should reflect problematic social behaviors (socially unacceptable behavior for the culture and community in which he/she lives) that put the child at some risk sanctions (e.g. not excessive shyness).

0 **Child shows no evidence of problematic social behaviors.**

1 **Mild level of problematic social behaviors. This might include occasionally inappropriate social behavior that forces adults to sanction the child. Infrequent inappropriate comments to strangers or unusual behavior in social settings might be included at this level.**

2 **Moderate level of problematic social behaviors. Social behavior is causing problems in the child's life. Child may be intentionally getting in trouble in school or at home.**

3 **Severe level of problematic social behaviors. This would be indicated by frequent seriously inappropriate social behavior that force adults to seriously and/or repeatedly sanction the child. Social behaviors are sufficiently severe that they place the child at risk of significant sanctions (e.g. expulsion, removal from the community).**

69. SEXUALLY REACTIVE BEHAVIORS

Sexually reactive behavior includes both age-inappropriate sexualized behaviors that may place a child at risk for victimization or risky sexual practices.

0 **No evidence of problems with sexually reactive behaviors or high-risk sexual behaviors.**

1 **Some evidence of sexually reactive behavior. Child may exhibit occasional inappropriate sexual language or behavior, flirts when age-inappropriate, or engages in unprotected sex with single partner. This behavior does not place child at great risk. A history of sexually provocative behavior would be rated here.**

2 **Moderate problems with sexually reactive behavior that place child at some risk. Child may exhibit more frequent sexually provocative behaviors in a manner that impairs functioning, engage in promiscuous sexual behaviors or have unprotected sex with multiple partners.**

3 **Significant problems with sexually reactive behaviors. Child exhibits sexual behaviors that place child or others at immediate risk.**

Ratings of Children Five Years Old and Younger

The following items are required for any child who is five years old or younger; however, they may be rated for any child if they represent a need for that specific individual.

70. MOTOR

This rating describes the child's fine (e.g. hand grasping and manipulation) and gross (e.g. sitting, standing, walking) motor functioning.

0 Child's fine and gross motor functioning appears normal. There is no reason to believe that the child has any problems with motor functioning.
1 The child has mild fine (e.g. using scissors) or gross motor skill deficits. The child may have exhibited delayed sitting, standing, or walking, but has since reached those milestones.
2 The child has moderate motor deficits. A non-ambulatory child with fine motor skills (e.g. reaching, grasping) or an ambulatory child with severe fine motor deficits would be rated here. A full-term newborn that does not have a sucking reflex in the first few days of life would be rated here.
3 The child has severe or profound motor deficits. A non-ambulatory child with additional movement deficits would be rated here, as would any child older than 6 months who cannot lift his or her head.

71. SENSORY

This rating describes the child's ability to use all senses including vision, hearing, smell, touch, and kinestetics.

0 The child's sensory functioning appears normal. There is no reason to believe that the child has any problems with sensory functioning.
1 The child has mild impairment on a single sense (e.g. mild hearing deficits, correctable vision problems).
2 The child has moderate impairment on a single sense or mild impairment on multiple senses (e.g. difficulties with sensory integration, diagnosed need for occupational therapy).
3 The child has significant impairment on one or more senses (e.g. profound hearing or vision loss).

72. COMMUNICATION

This rating describes the child's ability to communicate through any medium including all spontaneous vocalizations and articulations.

0 Child's receptive and expressive communication appears developmentally appropriate. There is no reason to believe that the child has any problems communicating.
1 Child's receptive abilities are intact, but child has limited expressive capabilities (e.g. if the child is an infant, he or she engages in limited vocalizations; if older than 24 months, he or she can understand verbal communication, but others have unusual difficulty understanding child).
2 Child has limited receptive and expressive capabilities.
3 Child is unable to communicate in any way, including pointing or grunting.

73. FAILURE TO THRIVE

Symptoms of failure to thrive focus on normal physical development such as growth and weight gain.

0 The child does not appear to have any problems with regard to weight gain or development. There is no evidence of failure to thrive.
1 The child has mild delays in physical development (e.g. is below the 25th percentile in terms of height or weight).
2 The child has significant delays in physical development that could be described as failure to thrive (e.g. is below the 10th percentile in terms of height or weight).
3 The child has severe problems with physical development that puts their life at risk (e.g. is at or beneath the 1st percentile in height or weight).

74. REGULATORY PROBLEMS

This category refer to all dimensions of self-regulation, including the quality and predictability of sucking/feeding, sleeping, elimination, activity level/intensity, sensitivity to external stimulation, and ability to be consoled.

0 Child does not appear to have any problems with self-regulation.
1 Child has mild problems with self-regulation (e.g. unusually intense activity level, mild or transient irritability).
2 Child has moderate to severe problems with self-regulation (e.g. chronic or intense irritability, unusually low tolerance/high sensitivity to external stimulation).
3 Child has profound problems with self-regulation that place his/her safety, well being, and/or development at risk (e.g. child cannot be soothed at all when distressed, child cannot feed properly).

75. BIRTH WEIGHT

This dimension describes the child's weight as compared to normal development.

0 **Child is within normal range for weight and has been since birth. A child with a birth weight of 2,500 g (5.5 pounds) or greater would be rated here.**
1 **Child was born under weight but is now within normal range or child is slightly beneath normal range. A child with a birth weight of between 1,500 g (3.3 pounds) and 2,499 g would be rated here.**
2 **Child is considerably under weight to the point of presenting a development risk to the child. A child with a birth weight of 1,000 ga (2.2 pounds) to 1,499 g would be rated here.**
3 **Child is extremely under weight to the point of the child's life is threatened. A child with a birth weight of less than 1,000 g (2.2 pounds) would be rated here.**

76. PICA

This item describes an eating disorder involving the compulsive ingestion of non-nutritive substances. Generally, the child must be older than 18 months to be considered with this problem.

0 **No evidence that the child eats unusual or dangerous materials.**
1 **Child has repeatedly eaten unusual or dangerous materials consistent with the diagnosis of Pica; however, this behavior has not occurred in the past 30 days.**
2 **Child has eaten unusual or dangerous materials consistent with the diagnosis of Pica in the past 30 days.**
3 **Child has become physically ill during the past 30 days by eating dangerous materials (e.g. lead paint).**

77. PRENATAL CARE

This dimension refers to the health care and birth circumstances experience by the child in utero.

0 **Child's biological mother had adequate prenatal care (e.g. ten or more planned visits to a physician) that began in the first trimester. Child's mother did not experience any pregnancy-related illnesses.**
1 **Child's mother had some short-comings in prenatal care, or had a mild form of a pregnancy-related illness. A child whose mother had six or fewer planned visits to a physician would be rated here (her care must have begun in the first or early second trimester). A child whose mother had a mild or well-controlled form of pregnancy-relayed illness such as gestational diabetes, or who had an uncomplicated high-risk pregnancy, would be rated here.**
2 **Child's biological mother received poor prenatal care, initiated only in the last trimester, or had a moderate form of pregnancy-related illness. A child whose mother had four or fewer planned visits to a physician would be rated**

here. A mother who experienced a high-risk pregnancy with some complications would be rated here.

3 Child's biological mother had no prenatal care, or had a severe form of pregnancy-related illness. A mother who had toxemia/pre-eclampsia would be rated here.

78. LABOR AND DELIVERY

This dimension refers to conditions associated with, and consequences arising from, complications in labor and delivery of the child.

0 Child and biological mother had normal labor and delivery. A child who received an Apgar score of 7–10 at birth would be rated here.

1 Child or mother had some mild problems during delivery, but child does not appear to be affected by these problems. An emergency C-Section or a delivery-related physical injury (e.g. shoulder displacement) to the child would be rated here.

2 Child or mother had problems during delivery that resulted in temporary functional difficulties for the child or mother. Extended fetal distress, post-partum hemorrhage, or uterine rupture would be rated here. A child who received an Apgar score of 4–7, or who needed some resuscitative measures at birth, would be rated here.

3 Child had severe problems during delivery that have long-term implications for development (e.g. extensive oxygen deprivation, brain damage). A child who received an Apgar score of 3 or lower, or who needed immediate or extensive resuscitative measures at birth, would be rated here.

79. SUBSTANCE EXPOSURE

This dimension describes the child's exposure to substance use and abuse both before and after birth.

0 Child had no in utero exposure to alcohol or drugs, and there is currently no exposure in the home.

1 Child had either mild in utero exposure (e.g. mother ingested alcohol or tobacco in small amounts fewer than four times during pregnancy), or there is current alcohol and/or drug use in the home.

2 Child was exposed to significant alcohol or drugs in utero. Any ingestion of illegal drugs during pregnancy (e.g. heroin, cocaine), or significant use of alcohol or tobacco, would be rated here.

3 Child was exposed to alcohol or drugs in utero and continues to be exposed in the home. Any child who evidenced symptoms of substance withdrawal at birth (e.g. crankiness, feeding problems, tremors, weak, and continual crying) would be rated here.

80. PARENT OR SIBLING PROBLEMS

This dimension describes how this child's parents and older siblings have done/are doing in their respective developments.

0 **The child's parents have no developmental disabilities. The child has no siblings, or existing siblings are not experiencing any developmental or behavioral problems**
1 **The child's parents have no developmental disabilities. The child has siblings who are experiencing some mild developmental or behavioral problems (e.g. Attention Deficit, Oppositional Defiant, or Conduct Disorders). It may be that child has at least one healthy sibling.**
2 **The child's parents have no developmental disabilities. The child has a sibling who is experiencing a significant developmental or behavioral problem (e.g. a severe version of any of the disorders cited above, or any developmental disorder).**
3 **One or both of the child's parents have been diagnosed with a developmental disability, or the child has multiple siblings who are experiencing significant developmental or behavioral problems (all siblings must have some problems).**

81. MATERNAL AVAILABILITY

This dimension addresses the primary caretaker's emotional and physical availability to the child in the weeks immediately following the birth. Rate maternal availability up until 3 months (12 weeks) post-partum.

0 **The child's mother/primary caretaker was emotionally and physically available to the child in the weeks following the birth.**
1 **The primary caretaker experienced some minor or transient stressors which made her slightly less available to the child (e.g. another child in the house under two years of age, an ill family member for whom the caretaker had responsibility, a return to work before the child reached six weeks of age).**
2 **The primary caretaker experienced a moderate level of stress sufficient to make him/her significantly less emotionally and physically available to the child in the weeks following the birth (e.g. major marital conflict, significant post-partum recuperation issues or chronic pain, two or more children in the house under four years of age).**
3 **The primary caretaker was unavailable to the child to such an extent that the child's emotional or physical well-being was severely compromised (e.g. a psychiatric hospitalization, a clinical diagnosis of severe Post-Partum Depression, any hospitalization for medical reasons which separated caretaker and child for an extended period of time, divorce or abandonment).**

82. CURIOUSITY

This rating describes the child's self-initiated efforts to discover his/her world.

0 This level indicates a child with exceptional curiosity. Infants display mouthing and banging of objects within grasp; older children crawl or walk to objects of interest.
1 This level indicates a child with good curiosity. An ambulatory child who does not walk to interesting objects, but who will actively explore them when presented to him/her, would be rated here.
2 This level indicates a child with limited curiosity. Child may be hesitant to seek out new information or environments, or reluctant to explore even presented objects.
3 This level indicates a child with very limited or no observable curiosity. Child may seem frightened of new information or environments.

83. PLAYFULNESS

This rating describes the child's enjoyment of play alone and with others.

0 This level indicates a child with substantial ability to play with self and others. Child enjoys play, and if old enough, regularly engages in symbolic and means-end play. If still an infant, child displays changing facial expressions in response to different play objects.
1 This level indicates a child with good play abilities. Child may enjoy play only with self or only with others, or may enjoy play with a limited selection of toys.
2 This level indicates a child with limited ability to enjoy play. Child may remain preoccupied with other children or adults to the exclusion of engaging in play, or may exhibit impoverished or unimaginative play.
3 This level indicates a child who has significant difficulty with play both by his/her self and with others. Child does not engage in symbolic or means-end play, although he or she will handle and manipulate toys.

Transition to Adulthood

The following items are required for youth 17 and older. However, any of these items can be rated regardless of age if they represent a need for a specific youth.

84. INDEPENDENT LIVING SKILLS

This rating focuses on the presence or absence of short or long-term risks associated with impairments in independent living abilities.

0 This level indicates a person who is fully capable of independent living. No evidence of any deficits that could impede maintaining own home.
1 This level indicates a person with mild impairment of independent living skills. Some problems exist with maintaining reasonable cleanliness, diet and so forth. Problems with money management may occur at this level. These problems are generally addressable with training or supervision.
2 This level indicates a person with moderate impairment of independent living skills. Notable problems with completing tasks necessary for independent living are apparent. Difficulty with cooking, cleaning, and self-management when unsupervised would be common at this level. Problems are generally addressable with in-home services.
3 This level indicates a person with profound impairment of independent living skills. This individual would be expected to be unable to live independently given their current status. Problems require a structured living environment.

85. TRANSPORTATION

This item is used to rate the level of transportation required to ensure that the individual could effectively participate in his/her own treatment and in other life activities. Only unmet transportation needs should be rated here.

0 The individual has no transportation needs.
1 The individual has occasional transportation needs (e.g., appointments). These needs would be no more than weekly and not require a special vehicle.
2 The individual has occasional transportation needs that require a special vehicle or frequent transportation needs (e.g., daily to work or therapy) that do not require a special vehicle.
3 The individual requires frequent (e.g., daily to work or therapy) transportation in a special vehicle.

86. PARENTING ROLES

This item is intended to rate the individual in any caregiver roles. For example, an individual with a son or daughter or an individual responsible for an elderly parent or grandparent would be rated here. Include pregnancy as a parenting role.

0 The individual has no role as a parent.
1 The individual has responsibilities as a parent but is currently able to manage these responsibilities.
2 The individual has responsibilities as a parent and either the individual is struggling with these responsibilities or they are currently interfering with the individual's functioning in other life domains.
3 The individual has responsibilities as a parent and the individual is currently unable to meet these responsibilities or these responsibilities are making it impossible for the individual to function in other life domains.

87. PERSONALITY DISORDER

This rating identifies the presence of any DSM-IV Axis II personality disorder

0 No evidence of symptoms of a personality disorder.
1 Evidence of mild degree, probably sub-threshold for the diagnosis of a personality disorder. For example, mild but consistent dependency in relationships might be rated here; or, some evidence of antisocial or narcissistic behavior. An unconfirmed suspicion of the presence of a diagnosable personality disorder would be rated here.
2 Evidence of sufficient degree of personality disorder to warrant a DSM-IV Axis II diagnosis.
3 Evidence of a severe personality disorder that has significant implications for the individual long-term functioning. Personality disorder dramatically interferes with the individuals ability to function independently.

88. INTIMATE RELATIONSHIPS

This item is used to rate the individuals current status in terms of romantic/intimate relationships.

0 Adaptive partner relationship. Individual has a strong, positive, partner relationship with another adult. This adult functions as a member of the family.
1 Mostly adaptive partner relationship. Individual has a generally positive partner relationship with another adult. This adult may not function as a member of the family.
2 Limited adaptive partner relationship. Individual is currently not involved in any partner relationship with another adult.
3 Significant difficulties with partner relationships. Individual is currently involved in a negative, unhealthy relationship with another adult.

89. MEDICATION COMPLIANCE

This rating focuses on the level of the individual's willingness and participation in taking prescribed medications.

0 This level indicates a person who takes any prescribed medications as prescribed and without reminders, or a person who is not currently on any psychotropic medication.
1 This level indicates a person who will take prescribed medications routinely, but who sometimes needs reminders to maintain compliance. Also, a history of medication noncompliance but no current problems would be rated here.
2 This level indicates a person who is somewhat non-compliant. This person may be resistant to taking prescribed medications or this person may tend to overuse his or her medications. He/she might comply with prescription plans for periods of time (1–2 weeks) but generally does not sustain taking medication in prescribed dose or protocol.

3 **This level indicates a person who has refused to take prescribed medications during the past 30 day period or a person who has abused his or her medications to a significant degree (i.e., overdosing or over using medications to a dangerous degree).**

90. EDUCATIONAL ATTAINMENT

This rates the degree to which the individual has completed his/her planned education.

0 **Individual has achieved all educational goals or has none but educational attainment has no impact on lifetime vocational functioning.**
1 **Individual has set educational goals and is currently making progress towards achieving them.**
2 **Individual has set educational goals but is currently not making progress towards achieving them.**
3 **Individual has no educational goals and lack of educational attainment is interfering with individual's lifetime vocational functioning.**

91. VICTIMIZATION

This item is used to examine a history and level of current risk for victimization.

0 **This level indicates a person with no evidence of recent victimization and no significant history of victimization within the past year. The person may have been robbed or burglarized on one or more occasions in the past, but no pattern of victimization exists. Person is not presently at risk for re-victimization.**
1 **This level indicates a person with a history of victimization but who has not been victimized to any significant degree in the past year. Person is not presently at risk for re-victimization.**
2 **This level indicates a person who has been recently victimized (within the past year) but is not in acute risk of re-victimization. This might include physical or sexual abuse, significant psychological abuse by family or friend, extortion, or violent crime.**
3 **This level indicates a person who has been recently victimized and is in acute risk of re-victimization. Examples include working as a prostitute and living in an abusive relationship.**

Caregiver Needs and Strengths

These ratings should be done focused on permanency plan caregivers. Caregiver ratings should be completed by household. If multiple households are involved in the permanency planning, then this section should be completed once for each household under consideration.

For Caregiver Needs and Strengths the following definitions and action levels apply:

0 indicates a dimension where there is no evidence of any needs. This is a strength
1 indicates a dimension that requires monitoring, watchful waiting, or preventive activities.
2 indicates a dimension that requires action to ensure that this identified need or risk behavior is addressed.
3 indicates a dimension that requires immediate or intensive action.

PHYSICAL HEALTH

Physical health includes medical and physical challenges faced by the caregiver(s)

0 Caregiver(s) has no physical health limitations that impact assistance or attendant care.
1 Caregiver(s) has some physical health limitations that interfere with provision of assistance or attendant care.
2 Caregiver(s) has significant physical health limitations that prevent them from being able to provide some needed assistance or make attendant care difficult.
3 Caregiver(s) is physically unable to provide any needed assistance or attendant care.

MENTAL HEALTH

This item refers to the caregiver's mental health status. Serious mental illness would be rated as a "2" or "3" unless the individual is in recovery.

0 Caregiver(s) has no mental health limitations that impact assistance or attendant care.
1 Caregiver(s) has some mental health limitations that interfere with provision of assistance or attendant care.
2 Caregiver(s) has significant mental health limitations that prevent them from being able to provide some needed assistance or make attendant care difficult.
3 Caregiver(s) is unable to provide any needed assistance or attendant care due to serious mental illness.

SUBSTANCE USE

This item rates the caregiver's pattern of alcohol and/or drug use. Substance-related disorders would be rated as a "2" or "3" unless the individual is in recovery.

0 Caregiver(s) has no substance-related limitations that impact assistance or attendant care.
1 Caregiver(s) has some substance-related limitations that interfere with provision of assistance or attendant care.

2 **Caregiver(s) has significant substance-related limitations that prevent them from being able to provide some needed assistance or make attendant care difficult.**
3 **Caregiver(s) is unable to provide any needed assistance or attendant care due to serious substance dependency or abuse.**

DEVELOPMENTAL

This item describes the caregiver's developmental status in terms of low IQ, mental retardation or other developmental disabilities.

0 **Caregiver(s) has no developmental limitations that impact assistance or attendant care.**
1 **Caregiver(s) has some developmental limitations that interfere with provision of assistance or attendant care.**
2 **Caregiver(s) has significant developmental limitations that prevent them from being able to provide some needed assistance or make attendant care difficult.**
3 **Caregiver(s) is unable to provide any needed assistance or attendant care due to serious developmental disabilities.**

SUPERVISION

This rating is used to determine the caregiver's capacity to provide the level of monitoring and discipline needed by the child.

0 **This rating is used to indicate a caregiver circumstance in which supervision and monitoring are appropriate and functioning well.**
1 **This level indicates a caregiver circumstance in which supervision is generally adequate but inconsistent. This may include a placement in which one member is capable of appropriate monitoring and supervision but others are not capable or not consistently available.**
2 **This level indicates a caregiver circumstance in which appropriate supervision and monitoring are very inconsistent and frequently absent.**
3 **This level indicates a caregiver circumstance in which appropriate supervision and monitoring are nearly always absent or inappropriate.**

INVOLVEMENT WITH CARE

This rating should be based on the level of involvement the caregiver(s) has in the planning and provision of child welfare and related services.

0 **This level indicates a caregiver(s) who is actively involved in the planning and/or implementation of services and is able to be an effective advocate on behalf of the child or adolescent.**

1 This level indicates a caregiver(s) who is consistently involved in the planning and/or implementation of services for the child or adolescent but is not an active advocate on behalf of the child or adolescent.
2 This level indicates a caregiver(s) who is minimally involved in the care of the child or adolescent. Caregiver may visit individual when in out of home placement, but does not become involved in service planning and implementation.
3 This level indicates a caregiver(s) who is uninvolved with the care of the child or adolescent. Caregiver may want individual out of home or fails to visit individual when in residential placement.

KNOWLEDGE

This rating should be based on caregiver's knowledge of the specific strengths of the child and any problems experienced by the child and their ability to understand the rationale for the treatment or management of these problems.

0 This level indicates that the present caregiver is fully knowledgeable about the child's psychological strengths and weaknesses, talents, and limitations.
1 This level indicates that the present caregiver, while being generally knowledgeable about the child, has some mild deficits in knowledge or understanding of either the child's psychological condition of his/her talents, skills, and assets.
2 This level indicates that the caregiver does not know or understand the child well and that significant deficits exist in the caregiver's ability to relate to the child's problems and strengths.
3 This level indicates that the present caregiver has little or no understanding of the child's current condition. The placement is unable to cope with the child given his/her status at the time, not because of the needs of the child but because the caregiver does not understand or accept the situation.

ORGANIZATION

This rating should be based on the ability of the caregiver to participate in or direct the organization of the household, services, and related activities.

0 Caregiver(s) is well organized and efficient.
1 Caregiver(s) has minimal difficulties with organizing or maintaining household to support needed services. For example, may be forgetful about appointments or occasionally fails to call back case manager.
2 Caregiver(s) has moderate difficulty organizing or maintaining household to support needed services.
3 Caregiver(s) is unable to organize household to support needed services.

RESOURCES

This item refers to the financial and social assets (extended family) and resources that the caregiver(s) can bring to bear in addressing the multiple needs of the child and family.

0 Caregiver(s) has sufficient resources so that there are few limitations on what can be provided for the child.
1 Caregiver(s) has the necessary resources to help address the child's major and basic needs but those resources might be stretched.
2 Caregiver(s) has limited resources (e.g. a grandmother living in same town who is sometimes available to watch the child).
3 Caregiver(s) has severely limited resources that are available to assist in the care and treatment of the child.

RESIDENTIAL STABILITY

This item rates the caregivers' current and likely future housing circumstances.

0 This rating indicates a family/caregiver in stable housing with no known risks of instability.
1 This rating indicates a family/caregiver that is currently in stable housing but there are significant risks of housing disruption (e.g. loss of job).
2 This rating indicates a family/caregiver that has moved frequently or has very unstable housing.
3 This rating indicates a family/caregiver that is currently homeless.

SAFETY

This rating refers to the safety of the assessed child. It does not refer to the safety of other family or household members based on any danger presented by the assessed child.

0 This level indicates that the present placement is as safe or safer for the child (in his or her present condition) as could be reasonably expected.
1 This level indicates that the present placement environment presents some mild risk of neglect, exposure to undesirable environments (e.g. drug use or gangs in neighborhood, etc.) but that no immediate risk is present.
2 This level indicates that the present placement environment presents a moderate level of risk to the child, including such things as the risk of neglect or abuse or exposure to individuals who could harm the child.
3 This level indicates that the present placement environment presents a significant risk to the well being of the child. Risk of neglect or abuse is imminent and immediate. Individuals in the environment offer the potential of significantly harming the child.

MARITAL/PARTNER VIOLENCE

This rating describes the degree of difficult or conflict in the caregiver relationship.

0 Caregivers appear to be functioning adequately. There is no evidence of notable conflict in the caregiver relationship. Disagreements are handled in an atmosphere of mutual respect and equal power.
1 Mild to moderate level of family problems including marital difficulties and caregiver arguments. Caregivers are generally able to keep arguments to a minimum when child is present. Occasional difficulties in conflict resolution or use of power and control by one partner over another.
2 Significant level of caregiver difficulties including frequent arguments that often escalate to verbal aggression or the use of verbal aggression by one partner to control the other. Child often witnesses these arguments between caregivers or the use of verbal aggression by one partner to control the other.
3 Profound level of caregiver or marital violence that often escalates to mutual attacks or the use of physical aggression by one partner to control the other. These episodes may exacerbate child's difficulties or put the child at greater risk.

CAREGIVER POSTTRAUMATIC REACTIONS

This rating describes posttraumatic reactions faced by caregiver(s), including emotional numbing and avoidance, nightmares, and flashbacks that are related to their child's or their own traumatic experiences.

0 Caregiver has adjusted to traumatic experiences without notable posttraumatic stress reactions.
1 Caregiver has some mild adjustment problems related to their child's or their own traumatic experiences. Caregiver may exhibit some guilt about their child's trauma or become somewhat detached or estranged from others.
2 Caregiver has moderate adjustment difficulties related to traumatic experiences. Caregiver may have nightmares or flashbacks of the trauma.
3 Caregiver has significant adjustment difficulties associated with traumatic experiences. Symptoms might include intrusive thoughts, hypervigilance, and constant anxiety.

PARENTAL CRIMINAL BEHAVIOR

This item rates the criminal behavior of both biological and stepparents.

0 There is no evidence that youth's parents have ever engaged in criminal behavior.
1 One of youth's parents has history of criminal behavior but youth has not been in contact with this parent for at least one year.
2 One of youth's parents has history of criminal behavior resulting in incarceration and youth has been in contact with this parent in the past year.
3 Both of youth's parents have history of criminal behavior resulting in incarceration.

Index

LaVergne, TN USA
02 February 2010
171864LV00002B/11/P

9 780387 928210